ENERGY MEDICINE YOGA

ENERGY MEDICINE YOGA

Amplify the Healing Power of Your Yoga Practice

LAUREN WALKER

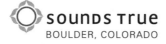

sounds true
BOULDER, COLORADO

Sounds True
Boulder, CO 80306

Sounds True is a trademark of Sounds True, Inc.

Cover design by Jennifer Miles
Book design by Beth Skelley

Printed in the United States of America

Library of Congress Cataloging-in-Publication Data
Walker, Lauren.
    Energy medicine yoga : amplify the healing power of your yoga practice / Lauren Walker.
      pages cm
    Includes bibliographical references.
    ISBN 978-1-62203-354-6 (alk. paper)
    1. Hatha yoga. 2. Energy medicine. I. Title.
    RA781.7.W345 2014
    613.7'046—dc23
                    2014011680

Ebook ISBN 978-1-62203-384-3

10 9 8 7 6 5 4 3 2 1

for Ricky and Rachel

CONTENTS

by Donna Eden

With its single three-word title, *Energy Medicine Yoga* manages to condense two very large domains—energy medicine and yoga. One of the root meanings of *yoga* is "to yoke," to combine, to form a union between two separate entities. In some renditions, this is thought of as achieving a union of *breath* and *body;* in others, of *body* and *consciousness;* in still others, of *human consciousness* and the *realm of divinity.* Moving to a quadruple entendre, the purpose of this book is also to create a yoga, a union of two disciplines that are usually practiced independently. I am honored to be asked to greet you on this journey into Energy Medicine Yoga by first putting energy medicine, as it pertains to this book, into context.

Albert Szent-Györgyi, a Nobel Laureate in Medicine, reflected that "in every culture and every medical tradition before ours, healing was accomplished by moving energy." Our culture is developing a thoroughly fresh approach to healing by reclaiming this ancient knowledge for working with the body's energies in a manner that is fully informed by modern scientific knowledge. Christiane Northrup, MD, explains: "In the medicine of the future, as I envision it, working with the patient's energy field will be the first intervention. Surgery will be a last resort. Drugs will be a last resort. They will still have their place, but shifting the energy patterns that caused the disease will be the first line of treatment." According to Stanford physicist William Tiller, "Modern medicine is rapidly approaching an age where energy will be considered the main factor in the diagnosis and treatment of disease." Mehmet Oz, MD, has famously suggested: "Energy medicine is the last great frontier in medicine."

Because there are already so many approaches to energy medicine, and this book focuses on the one with which I am associated, I need to begin by sharing a bit about how I came to the methods I use. My approach to energy medicine actually grew out of a series of personal health challenges. I was born with vulnerabilities that resulted in asthma and severe allergies. I contracted tuberculosis at age three and was diagnosed with multiple sclerosis at sixteen. As my body deteriorated and my organs began to break down, I had a heart attack at twenty-seven and was not expected to live beyond my early thirties. Nonetheless, I had a few things going for me. I had managed to birth two beautiful daughters by my mid-twenties, and I had a natural attunement to the subtle energies in the human body, able to see and sense them in myself and in others.

After several doctors told me to get my "affairs in order," my determination to not leave my daughters joined with my facility with energy, driving me to figure out the steps I needed to take to heal myself. In bed and often unable to walk, I focused on where the energies in my body seemed stuck or painful and devised ways to soothe those energies and get them moving. To everyone's surprise, I grew stronger and healthier after medical avenues had been abandoned. By my mid-thirties, I was in the best health of my life, and I wanted to aid others who were suffering from serious illnesses. This became the guiding purpose of my life.

Only after I had become involved in the health challenges of those who sought my help did I begin to study the healing traditions of other cultures. I learned that the body's energies have been mapped by many systems, and I was fascinated to discover that these maps often correspond with the way I see energies moving when a client is on my table.

Three systems that stood out for me were 1) the Celtic healing arts that had been passed down orally and with which I had an intuitive connection, 2) drawings and descriptions of energy pathways by ancient Chinese physicians, and 3) yoga techniques and principles that have been practiced for millennia. In yoga are found postures (*asanas*) and breathing techniques (*pranayama*) to restore, maintain, and direct the vital energies of the life force. Fused with these practices were descriptions of vortexes of energy, called *chakras,* and channels along which energy flows, called *nadis,* both of which I could see and had been regulating with my clients.

I began to call the method I was developing "energy medicine," realizing that it was not so much a new system but rather another approach for working with the same vital energies that had been the focus of many healing and spiritual traditions before it. One of my students, the author of this book, was already an accomplished yoga practitioner and teacher, and she began integrating methods I was teaching her into her yoga practice. When I learned of this, I became very interested to see how she was approaching it. Now after having read this book, I am extraordinarily impressed with the synthesis she has created.

Yoga is, of course, among the oldest existing systems for enhancing the health of the body's energy systems. Since my approach to working with the body's energies grew out of overcoming my own maladies, it addresses physical illness in ways that are much more focused than a typical yoga routine. It includes strategies for assessing the performance of every organ and every other system of the body, healing their disorders, and optimizing their functioning. Through my clients and students, I have learned that these methods are valuable not only for overcoming illness but also for maintaining health and increasing vitality.

In marrying energy medicine techniques with time-honored yoga postures and positions, Lauren Walker has created a brilliant system that draws on the strengths of each discipline, and you are the beneficiary. *Energy Medicine Yoga* teaches you a basic yoga routine. But every step of the way—from warm-up to cool-down—is interlaced with specific techniques that enhance the physical and mental benefits of the posture. Whether you are a beginner learning both energy medicine and yoga from the book, a seasoned yoga practitioner wanting to bring the benefits of energy medicine into your routines, or already proficient in energy medicine and interested in combining its benefits with the benefits of yoga, this work is a powerful resource.

I asked Lauren how she had the gumption to try to improve on a system that had been revered by generation after generation for thousands of years. She told me that as her own footing as a yoga teacher was developing, she started taking classes from some of the most well-known yoga teachers and began to look at their impact on students through the perspective she had cultivated during her energy medicine training. From that vantage point, she felt that their classes "weren't shifting the students' energies except at the most basic level." Even a yoga class that "exhausts you or exhilarates you," she told me, "doesn't work with the underlying energy levels." So she set out to intro- duce energy medicine into her own yoga practice to accomplish this, and she has succeeded magnificently.

The core of the book presents an eight-week program that teaches you, a week at a time, specific sets of postures and energy medicine skills which, in week 8, are mercifully woven together into a daily practice that can be done in a mere twenty minutes. Energy medicine is not a simple discipline to master. The body has multiple energy systems. You are familiar with some of them, such as the chakras, aura, and meridians, but others such as the radiant circuits and Celtic

Weave have not made it into our common vocabulary. Lauren breaks down this complexity by introducing a new system (or two or three) each week and showing you concrete benefits of working with that system.

The book is, in fact, laced with detailed ways that energy medicine techniques can enhance a yoga practice. I'll mention only a few. *Energy Medicine Yoga* begins with a two-minute "Wake-up" routine to get your energies "moving in the right direction" so that you will already be in a flow when you begin the physical postures. Because yoga stretches you—literally and figuratively—you come up against pain, tension, or soreness when you are doing the practices correctly. Lauren teaches an energy medicine technique that works with reflex points that get the body's energies moving in areas where they are congealed. Such congealed energies are a major cause of your body's daily aches and pains. If you clear them before your yoga stretches, you have made space for the energy to flow so the stretch can go a bit further and with a bit less tenderness. That is the cat's meow as your yoga practice advances. Another area where energy medicine and yoga team up nicely involves emotions that may emerge during a yoga practice. Yoga teachers are well aware that different parts of the body may hold memories or emotions that can be released during yoga postures. The back may hold feelings of being weighted down. The hips may hold unresolved sexual feelings. While the release of these feelings may be cathartic, they may also be overwhelming and persist long after the yoga session. Lauren teaches you another set of reflex points used in energy medicine that can be applied when unexpected emotion or the residue of past trauma is released and you are left feeling agitated and unresolved.

Throughout *Energy Medicine Yoga,* you will also find some of the clearest and most concrete metaphors I've ever seen in a book that addresses the body's energies. Lauren is an avid skier, and the book opens by taking us on a ski-lift ride to survey the groomed ski runs below. The tracks of the skiers are smoothed each night so they don't become deep ruts that can't be skied. "This daily process of tracking up and then grooming the mountain is not unlike how the energies of the body work," Lauren explains. "The ski runs are the body's energy systems, and the skiers are all the processes that track up the systems. Every single thing we do—digest food, move, think, talk—takes the body out of neutral and tips its delicate balance. The body is then always trying to get back into balance, just as the groomers are always trying to keep the slopes groomed. Losing, regaining, and maintaining that balance—the homeostasis of the body—is the dance of being alive."

Energy Medicine Yoga gives you a system that, in twenty minutes each day, can help support your body's ability to stay in balance. Whether you read it to learn more about yoga, to learn more about energy medicine, or to adopt the powerful practices it presents into your daily life, you will, for your efforts, have become a better skier of your body's energies.

Donna Eden
April 23, 2014
Ashland, Oregon

What Is Energy Medicine Yoga?

"What exactly *is* Energy Medicine Yoga?" Jen asked, as we pulled down the safety bar on the chairlift and started our seven-minute ascent. She had already signed up for my "Introduction to Energy Medicine Yoga" series, because she said I was her favorite yoga teacher and she'd take any class I offered. But it'd been ten years since I'd lived in Montana and taught here, and my teaching had evolved significantly since then. Jen had no idea what I was going to offer.

"You can give me the elevator pitch," she said. "Or the chairlift pitch."

We were rising up the mountain and could see the groomed ski runs beneath us. Every day, as soon as the chairlifts close, huge machines come out and groom the slopes. They smooth out all the imprints made by the skiers, they pull snow that has been pushed to the edges back to the middle of the runs, and they take newly fallen snow and set all of that down in corduroy patterns. They work all night long, until the entire mountain is organized, clean, and set in neat, smooth runs. Then, when the first chairlifts open, the skiers and snowboarders descend and start tracking up the mountain again. The whole cycle repeats, day after day.

This daily process of tracking up and then grooming the mountain is not unlike how the energies of the body work, I explained to Jen. The ski runs are the body's energy systems, and the skiers are all the processes that track up the systems. Every single thing we do—digest food, move, think, talk—takes the body out of neutral and tips its delicate balance. The body is then always trying to get back into balance, just as the groomers are always trying to keep the slopes groomed. Losing, regaining, and maintaining that balance—the homeostasis of the body—is the dance of being alive.

When the body is healthy, it is able to easily rebalance itself. Even when something extreme happens—we break a leg or catch the flu—the body can deal with it, heal it, and come back to center. But when the energies of the body are stressed for too long, they start to stay in an unbalanced place, and it becomes harder and harder for the body to heal or come to neutral.

If one of the grooming machines on the mountain is out of service, all the other groomers have to work harder to get the mountain ready for opening. Some of the runs don't get groomed, and they get less and less skiable. The tracks become huge, deep moguls, and fewer people have the skill to ski these damaged runs. The same thing happens to our bodies' energies. Consistent imbalances lead to chronic problems like adrenal fatigue, depression, lingering illness, and a general feeling of being unwell or off in some hard-to-name, but certain way.

Our mountain has always been known for its amazing groomed runs. The best groomer operators are the ones who have a deep intimacy with the mountain. They know every bump and rise, fall line, tree line. They know where there is extra snow they can pull from, where there are bare or rough areas that need attention. They know where to open up side trails to connect main runs when the crowds get too big. They know the spots that get habitually scraped of snow, and the ones that get clogged with excess snow. They spend hours and hours massaging and clearing the landscape, and the best operators feel a singular love for the snowfields. The very best ones—and these are a rare few—know the mountain in all its seasons. They know which trees and shrubs should be cut back in summer, and they are often the ones to cut them back, to help clear debris. They build culverts and ditches for the spring runoff so the slopes don't erode. They build biking and hiking trails for the way people move around the mountain in the spring, summer, and fall. They know how to work with all the elements at play on these fields. In much the same way, we want to create an intimacy with our own bodies. We want to know where there is excess energy, where there are lacks, how to move and direct the energy, clear barriers, widen pathways—in all the different seasons.

Energy Medicine Yoga is essentially grooming the body's energies, the way the operators groom the snow on the mountain. It helps us make sure the body's energies are awake and moving, that they are running forward and not backward (a very common occurrence), and that the energy systems of the body are coordinated and organized. Some of the energy systems require clearing, like blowing out a kitchen drain blocked by grease. Some of them require holding and rocking, like calming a screaming baby. Some of them require gentle tapping and smoothing, like puttying over a hole in a wall. Some of them require deep-pressure massage, like pressing a ball of pie dough into a pie tin. Some of them require weaving together, like darning a hole in a sock.

I promised Jen that in our eight-week Energy Medicine Yoga class, she would learn what these energy systems of the body are and how to easily take care of them. She would learn how to develop her own daily, twenty- to forty-minute Energy Medicine Yoga practice that would allow her to feel strong, balanced, and stress free no matter what was going on in her life. Her physical body would feel more easeful and recover better both from her workouts and the challenges of having three small children. And her mind would be able to digest her experiences and help her identify and achieve her goals, both professional and spiritual.

"That's a lot to promise," she said, with a glint in her eye.

I agreed, but I was also confident. I knew from my own experience that if the body's energies are balanced, if they have space and room to move, and if they are being supported by intelligent practices, there is nothing we can't handle. Combining the two powerful paradigms of yoga and energy medicine had helped me shift out of some deeply embedded and unsatisfying patterns that were holding me back and draining my energy. And as I've taught Energy Medicine Yoga to others, many of my students have told me they were able to do the same things.

At the military college where I taught for four years, most people knew about yoga. Even if they thought of it as just stretching, they had some idea, because yoga has infiltrated the mainstream. To a T, those with limited knowledge were blown away by how Energy Medicine Yoga helped them to release stress, to get more done in their days, and to succeed in their goals in a more easeful way. They also commented on how their relationships improved. They thought they would stretch, which they did. But they did not know that they would learn how to breathe, how their bodies worked, how their minds worked, and how to change both the body and the mind with a directed, intelligent, and easy-to-learn practice.

Every yoga book will tell you that the word *yoga* itself means "union"—literally, "to yoke," to bring two disparate things together. In the yoga context, this initially means bringing together movements of the breath and the body. Later, as you go deeper in the yoga practices, it means bringing together the body and the mind.

But as I was writing this introduction, I found in one of my notebooks from the many workshops I've taken with my yoga teacher, Rod Stryker, a definition that held much more meaning. *Yoga,* in its ultimate context, means to merge with that part of us that is unchanging, universal, and omniscient. Yoga is a science both of being and of becoming, and how I, as the practitioner, can influence the direction of change. It helps us to answer the constant question, "What next?"

That understanding of yoga is at the heart of Energy Medicine Yoga: it is the practice of influencing the direction of our body's energy patterns in order to create positive change.

Energy medicine is prevalent in our world, and encompasses many different paradigms. Acupuncture, tai chi, ultrasound, Reiki, magnetic resonance imaging (MRI), laser surgery, and radiation therapy are all forms of energy medicine. But the model of energy medicine that we'll follow in this book comes from my energy medicine teacher, Donna Eden: "Energy medicine is the art and science of fostering physical, psychological, and spiritual health and wellbeing. It combines a rational knowledge and intuitive understanding of the energies in the body and in the environment. . . . By focusing on your body as a living system of energy, you begin to realize that powerful energy technologies are *already* inherent in your hands and in your being."

Energy, for our purpose, is the capacity to perform work and an internal power used to produce an effect. In Energy Medicine Yoga, we use the power of energy, aligned with its healing principles, to harness our own life force and both transform ourselves to our highest good and accept ourselves in our innate perfection.

Energy Medicine Yoga is designed to teach you to communicate with your body the way your body can understand. This is a two-way street. Our bodies, and souls, talk to us in numerous ways. Messages come to us through our dreams, intuitions, and feelings, as well as through physical sensations like pleasure and pain. We need to learn to speak back to our bodies on a deeper level, in the same language that the body itself speaks. We do this in a variety of ways: through imagination, visualization, meditation, and through physical means such as touching, tapping, holding specific points, stretching, and massage.

Part of the development of Energy Medicine Yoga came from my time teaching at Norwich University, the oldest private military college in the country. As I saw the effects this practice had on the men and women preparing to serve our country, I determined that I wanted to offer it to as many deploying soldiers as possible. Using the template of the eight-week basic training that every soldier undergoes, I designed a program to give these Energy Medicine Yoga tools to people about to face some of the most intensely stressful situations possible.

The eight-week course also turned out to be the best way to teach both beginner and advanced yoga students in the same setting. People who had never heard of *bandhas* learned them, along with the important yoga postures. Advanced students and yoga teachers were able to greatly increase the power of their existing practice by incorporating Energy Medicine Yoga techniques into it, while also learning how to apply the energy medicine principles to the yoga basics. The eight-week course I developed at Norwich became the template for the series of eight-week workshops I now teach at yoga studios around the United States, and forms the framework for this book.

This work is derived from my intensive studies with two teachers. Rod Stryker, who created ParaYoga, has been my teacher since 2000 and has taught me more than I ever imagined yoga could encompass. He also encouraged me to keep teaching when I was close to quitting yoga altogether. Donna Eden, the founder of Eden Energy Medicine, came into my life when it was at a serious low point, and she helped to spark the radiant circuits that started to fill me with joy again. Being welcomed into her family of students and teachers and studying her system of energy medicine transformed my life.

The incredible wisdom and knowledge of these two master teachers form the basis of Energy Medicine Yoga: a modern tantra, or weaving, of ancient wisdom to help us heal and thrive.

Because the organization of the book mirrors the layout of my eight-week course series, you can use part 1 as your own personal eight-week Energy Medicine Yoga workshop. Spending a week with each of the chapters in part 1 before moving on to the next is a great way to become familiar with Energy Medicine Yoga and build a practice of your own. If you already have a yoga practice that works for you, you can read through part 1 and pull different Energy Medicine Yoga practices out of each section and insert them directly into what you already do, empowering the poses with the simple techniques. You can also just try doing a pose here or there to start to learn what Energy Medicine Yoga is all about.

Part 1 lays the groundwork for your Energy Medicine Yoga practice, including key energy systems of the body and other basic concepts. It gives you a wealth of powerful practices and, at the end, shows you how they can become a twenty- to forty-minute Energy Medicine Yoga routine.

That template is a map you will use to chart your course through part 2, which gives you additional Energy Medicine Yoga practices that I've discovered or developed—dozens of poses you can add to the basic template. For example, you can add standing poses into the Energy Medicine Yoga sun salutation or directly after it, and you can add more twists or forward bends at the appropriate place in your practice.

Throughout this book, you'll see many Sanskrit words. Sanskrit, an ancient language with roots in India, is the language of yoga, and though you may not have seen these words before, you've probably heard your yoga teacher say them. Many yoga teachers, myself included, use both the Sanskrit and English names for poses and practices—sometimes together, sometimes interchangeably. Sanskrit is a resonant language, which means it has the subtle but real effect of opening up energy pathways in the body as the words themselves are spoken. Using Sanskrit is also the traditional way of teaching yoga. Out of respect and love for these ancient roots, Sanskrit is used (and translated) liberally throughout this text.

Energy Medicine Yoga does not rely heavily on props, so whatever props you generally use for your yoga practice are all that is needed here. A mat, a blanket, and one or two blocks would be helpful. A strap is good to have but not necessary.

If you've never practiced yoga before, you will certainly be able to do the practices laid out here, but the focus of this book is weaving these energy techniques into your established yoga practice and into poses you already know. Though I will take you through the basics and build each pose from the toes up, this book is not all about alignment. If you have never practiced yoga before, I suggest taking a class at your local studio or gym or watching some beginner-level videos. If you've practiced yoga even only a few times, or if you are a yoga teacher with years of experience, the techniques here will help transform what you've been doing and help you take your yoga to new, dynamic, and exciting places.

I invite you to dive in and find your own path through the amazing and beautiful fields of energy in your own body!

Starting Your Energy Medicine Yoga Practice

Here in part 1, you will learn everything you need to know for an effective Energy Medicine Yoga practice. The first seven weeks will introduce many new concepts and poses. If you're familiar with yoga, the poses and practices will seem like strange variations on those you already do. If you're new to yoga, these practices will be your baseline. The poses are what I call the essentials or the power poses—the ones that give you the most bang for your buck. If you have only a short time, or your body just needs maintenance, or if you're traveling or recovering from a strain, injury, or illness, these poses are your go-to poses.

Each chapter of part 1 also offers concepts to take you deeper—to add even more power to the poses, help you discover and strengthen your own energy field, and start to learn how your unique energy works. Week 8 will help you tie together all the concepts and practices from weeks 1 through 7 into an ideal, twenty- to forty-minute Energy Medicine Yoga practice. This template can be your whole practice, because it is complete and comprehensive and serves well as a daily routine. It can also serve as the basis for a longer practice, as you'll learn in part 2.

All practices in Energy Medicine Yoga work with the underlying energy systems of your body. These energy systems come from many different healing traditions. The chakras are yogic or Vedic from Indian culture; the meridians and radiant circuits go back to Traditional Chinese Medicine (TCM). Each tradition has its own way of describing similar energetic phenomena, and the two oldest medicines on the planet, Ayurveda (the yogic health system) and TCM, overlap both in the holistic way they look at the body and in the treatments they provide.

Each energy system is a discrete, complete system, and they all interconnect and interrelate. They affect and are affected by each other. They also reflect and are reflected back by the health of the physical body. Like the systems of the body in Western medicine (such as the skeletal, nervous, lymphatic, circulatory, and muscular systems), these systems of energy are integral unto themselves yet also influence each other.

Each week/chapter, I introduce one to three of the energy systems of the body and share practices that get these systems and their energies working well for you. Keep in mind that it takes longer to read the practice directions than to actually do them! Once you take the instructions to your mat and start doing them, you'll see firsthand how naturally energy medicine techniques blend into your yoga poses. And once you see the impact these practices have on your overall energy, you'll wonder how you ever did yoga without them.

Welcome to Energy Medicine Yoga

In our increasingly busy world, where the things pulling our attention are myriad and never ending, we have limited time to do a practice to keep ourselves healthy and balanced both spiritually and physically. So rather than ask you to add one more thing to your already busy lives, I propose following the military adage of working "smarter not harder."

Once you learn what energy means in the body and how to work with it, you'll see how so much of your time is spent fighting against yourself. Like rowing a boat upstream, you often work harder than you need to, to get to where you want to go. The goal with Energy Medicine Yoga is to turn the boat around, so you are flowing easily with the currents of energy that are already working in your body. When you do this, you will also be able to harness that energy to use how you need it, like the power of a well-placed power-generating dam.

Most of us experience energy in only the most pedestrian of ways: we feel tired or full of energy. Those two ends of the spectrum seem to be our only way of expressing how we experience energy's effects on us. Unlike the Inuit, who have more than two dozen words for snow, we have woefully few words to explain that which is essentially the underpinning fact of life itself.

Energy medicine gives us a more detailed and complete, but also very simple, explanation of how energy works, specifically in relation to our physical bodies. It teaches us that:

Energy wants to move and needs space to move.
Energy moves in patterns. There are specific and easily definable patterns of energy within and around the physical body that are always the same. Once you learn these patterns, you can help balance and strengthen the energy running along their pathways.

Energy forms habits. Energy not only runs in patterns, but also forms habits. These habits are not always beneficial. The good news is that energy can be repatterned, and energy medicine techniques help you do this.

Energy has priorities, and these priorities are consistent. The first priority of energy in your body is to keep you alive. Your energy keeps the essential physical systems of your body functioning and healthy, sometimes sacrificing less important systems to do so. After that, your energies support your intentions, both conscious and unconscious. For example, if the body's energies are busy healing your physical form, they are not available to help you fulfill your desire for a new job.

Energy is affected by thoughts, environment, and the people we come into contact with. By changing any of these, you can change your energy flow and, therefore, your life. Because energy is also deeply affected by the people around you and by your environment, an important means of improving your personal energy landscape is to remove yourself from toxic people and from a toxic environment. This change becomes even more critical if you are unwell.

Once I started learning about energy medicine from Donna Eden, some of the things that hadn't made sense to me before started to, such as how it was so easy to shift and move certain energetic patterns of the body by simply waving your hands around, tapping here, and smoothing out some skin there. I also began to understand how some energetic patterns are deeply embedded and, thus, hard to shift.

These patterns or habits are actually energy fields. An energy field is like a body of water: There are many things happening on the surface and in the depths. There are ecosystems that live within the field of the water; there are schools of many different species of fish, as well as aquatic plant life and microorganisms. Each of these forms its own system, and together, they form the field of the body of water. If you change any one of the components, the entire ecosystem changes. When you drop a rock into the water, ripples of energy move through the field. These ripples follow certain laws of physics, just as energy does, and affect the field of the body of water, but the ripples are also their own energetic event. When you realize how you can change the whole field by changing one component, you start to see how interrelated everything truly is. The same is true of our personal energy fields: they are all interrelated, and when you change one component of one of your energy systems, you also affect all the other systems. When that knowledge is coupled with very specific tools, miracles really can happen.

Often energy gets stuck in one specific location or fixed in patterns. This stuck or fixed energy becomes painful, and that pain signifies that something, whether it is physical or emotional, needs to move. Like water getting stuck behind a fallen tree in a river, the energy has to change its direction to get around the impediment. Sometimes the logjam becomes so large that the water/energy actually turns and heads back upstream. Or it builds up into a deep and stagnant pool, waiting for another force of nature to remove the obstacle. Or the buildup causes the river of energy to flood its banks, affecting the entire surrounding area.

Energy starts out in its subtlest form and moves toward its densest form. And when it gets dense and slows down, it is going against the first two principles outlined earlier: energy needs to move, and energy needs space to move. In Donna Eden's system of energy medicine, all pathologies can essentially be traced back to the need to move energy and to give it space to do so. The primary reason Energy Medicine Yoga is so powerful is that we are taking the densest energy, our physical form, and opening up space within it so that our more subtle energies can also move.

When you first begin to practice Energy Medicine Yoga, you'll probably be asking yourself, how does the energy move and what does it feel like? As soon as you start to feel pulses under your hands, energy starts to be less theoretical and more visceral. You actually feel energies moving, coming alive, reorganizing in your body, in a way you may never have before. Every time my energetic pulses synch up when I'm doing a meridian treatment, for example, I'm astonished anew at how powerful they are. Trust the wisdom of your body.

Waking Up the Body's Energies

This week you'll learn how energy works in the body and how to wake it up. I'll show you how to explore this energy using the body's own language.

Energy System of the Week: The Meridians

The meridian system is one of the most well-known and most-used energy systems in the Western world, having the advantage of acupuncture as its primary ambassador. The meridians transport energy through the body similar to the way that veins and arteries carry blood. They are specific pathways that run in the same consistent patterns in every body. These pathways run deep in the body and then come close to the skin at several points. It is these surface points that are used in acupressure and acupuncture and that we'll use in Energy Medicine Yoga.

There are eleven main meridians, each of which corresponds to a different organ and feeds energy to that respective organ: liver, lung, large intestine, stomach, spleen, heart, small intestine, bladder, kidney, circulation-sex (pericardium), and gallbladder. The twelfth meridian, the triple warmer, does not correspond to a specific organ, but relates to three areas of the body and has its hand in many of the functions of the body. Because of its enormous role and power, it is also considered its own energy system; we'll explore the triple warmer system in more detail in week 4. Two other meridians, the central and governing meridians, run vertically around the core of the body. The meridians are actually all connected and form one long, continuous path of energy through the body.

The meridians can be closely correlated to the nadis of yoga, which are also energy pathways. In Ayurveda and many traditions of yoga, there are fourteen major nadis (some traditions cite thirteen). Each of the nadis starts at the base of the spine, at the *kanda,* where the coiled potential energy (commonly referred to as *kundalini*) is located. The nadis run in pairs parallel to the spine, connect to a chakra, and then distribute that chakra energy to the body. It's interesting that in both TCM and yoga there are fourteen major energetic paths in the body.

Each meridian is either yin or yang in nature. The concept of yin and yang is extremely important in Energy Medicine Yoga. It is the idea of opposites in a constant dance of balance. These forces, both opposing and complementary, exist in everything—night and day, light and dark, masculine and feminine. They are the dynamic interplay of the universal forces that give rise to existence. Everything contains both yin and yang. The balance comes from the continuing cycle of life. The expression "It is always darkest before the dawn" is a perfect representation of the yin-yang symbol, which has the big tadpole head turn instantly into the tiny point of the tail that then leads back to the head. The yin gets smaller and smaller and smaller until it becomes the smallest point, and at that moment, it bursts into its biggest opposite. Then it slowly diminishes again, smaller and smaller, until it is a point, and then it becomes enormous again. That's the cycle, around and around.

All the different processes of life also follow this same circular, yin-yang cycle of both balancing and transforming. Life is like a gyroscope, not a still point. All of the processes at work in our bodies spin and transform, and sometimes they have wobbles in them. They spin, and sometimes they slow, but they always continue to transform from yin to yang and back again. That spinning from yin to yang is the perpetual energy of life. When those energies get stuck or slow (the wobble), you have to help move the energy along its path. Energy Medicine Yoga—or acupuncture or another type of energy work—can be the intervention needed to help the energy move smoothly again.

Yin meridians flow upward—up the front or inside of the body and out from the chest on the soft inside of the arms to the hands. Yin energy flows up from the earth, inward, deep and inside the body. Forces of yin are feminine energies—receptive, yielding, and inward. They are associated with the moon, water, cold, dark, night, autumn, winter.

Yang meridians flow down the front, back, or outside of the body. They flow from the back of the hands toward the torso, along the outside of the arms to the face, and down the back of the body. They move outward and govern our action in the world. Yang forces come down from the heavens and are the masculine energies—active, assertive, outward directed. They are the energies of the sun, fire, heat, light, day, spring, summer.

In Energy Medicine Yoga, we work with the directions of the meridians in a more general and unifying way. If you want to know the exact path of each meridian, Donna Eden's book *Energy Medicine* offers great illustrations. There are also websites with diagrams and specific meridian-point locaters. I like Acupuncture.com and Yin Yang House (yinyanghouse.com) the best.

Other Important Concepts: Reflex Points

There are a few other key things to know as we get started with the practices for week 1.

NEUROLYMPHATIC REFLEX POINTS

These are points on the body that, when pressed and massaged deeply, trigger the lymph to dump its debris into the venous blood supply for elimination from the body. The lymph system, which is responsible for detoxing the body, does not have its own pump. It relies on ancillary movement of the body to pump it through its vessels. A practice like yoga is helpful for moving lymph, but often it isn't enough.

When a doctor taps a hammer on your knee, a reflex is triggered, and your foot kicks forward. Similarly, when you deeply massage neurolymphatic reflex points, a reflex is triggered in the corresponding organ, and that organ releases its lymph into the venous blood. It may be uncomfortable or painful to press these points deeply, but releasing the stagnant energy and toxins makes the discomfort worth it. Working these points also helps to get meridian energy moving to start the healing process.

Releasing toxins (detoxing) via the lymphatic system can make you tired or even feel ill, depending on how toxic your system is. Go slowly, working the neurolymphatic reflex points a little bit each day instead of trying to work all of them hard at once. It can be helpful to take a saltwater bath after working with these points, to help support the cleansing process.

NEUROVASCULAR REFLEX POINTS

These points connect the nervous system and circulatory system with the meridians and their elements. (For more about the five elements and their meridian correspondences, see week 5.) Holding or massaging the neurovascular reflex points directs blood flow, hormone movement, and energetic patterns to calm and stabilize the nervous system, which helps to end the emergency-response loop. Because of these effects, massaging and holding these points helps train your brain to stay calm in the face of thoughts, feelings, circumstances, and danger, real or imagined.

These points also correspond to different organs in the body. When held, they bring increased blood flow to those organs, as well as help to disperse and release the emotional energy connected with the organ. When massaged, they wake up and start to release their excess energy, especially if they are sore and you give them extra attention.

When simply holding these points, a light touch is used, because you're stimulating the capillary beds so that blood returns to and stays in the forebrain. When the forebrain has enough blood, discernment and creative thinking are possible during a stressful situation; the physical responses of fleeing or fighting are triggered when the blood leaves the forebrain.

Working these points also helps balance the meridians, and because the meridians are associated with different emotions, these points are very powerful tools for working with the emotions.

Pranayama (Breathing Practices): Energy Medicine Yoga Breath Versus Regular Yoga Breath

In most yoga classes, the instructions are to breathe in and out through the nose. This type of breathing helps contain and build energy. It is also a form of biofeedback that shows you where you are in your yoga practice; if the physical work gets too challenging, the breath rate increases, and you may have to open your mouth to let more oxygen in. But breathing through your mouth incites a stress response, the exact opposite of what you're hoping to achieve with yoga. So instead of defaulting to a mouth breath to meet the physical demands, you regulate and slow down the physical practice. As you get stronger in your practice and build lung capacity, you are able to work harder physically while still maintaining a nose-breathing pattern.

In energy medicine, you breathe in through the nose and out through the mouth. This breathing helps to facilitate and reinforce the connection between the central and governing meridians—the core energies on the trunk of the body. They connect where the hard and soft palate meet at the top and back of the mouth. If you sit still and breathe just once in through your nose and out through your mouth, you can feel a circle with the breath. You feel the breath coming in the nose, and when you exhale through the mouth, you physically feel the breath, at the top of the mouth. The in breath *touches* the out breath here. This type of breathing is also the breathing used in the Taoist meditation known as the microcosmic orbit, which is a meditation and visualization technique for cycling energy through the body.

Another important reason to exhale through the mouth is that it releases excess energy. During an Energy Medicine Yoga practice (or any yoga practice, for that matter), as you move stuck energy, you may feel overwhelmed by emotion. A way to facilitate the release of that emotion from the body is to exhale through the mouth.

As you spend more time in your Energy Medicine Yoga practice, you'll start to build the knowledge and intelligence needed to know when a mouth exhale is necessary or when to slow down the physical work to maintain a nose breath.

For the Wake Up, the opening sequence of techniques in any Energy Medicine Yoga practice, you'll breathe in through the nose and out through the mouth. As you move on, you'll adopt the yogic breath of in the nose, out the nose. As you start to tune in to your practice, watch your breath. It will become one of your greatest teachers.

Practices of the Week: The Wake Up

The first step of your Energy Medicine Yoga practice is to awaken the body and get all its energies moving in the right direction. Just as your computer has a power button and your car has an ignition switch, the body has its own set of buttons and switches for waking it up. These four techniques come directly from the Daily Energy Routine that Donna Eden teaches and that appears in her book *Energy Medicine*. Her daily routine has many more elements than just these four, but I took the four that were the most important in terms of starting your yoga practice.

The Wake Up encompasses four energy medicine techniques to be done at the beginning of any Energy Medicine Yoga practice. These simple exercises—the Four Thumps, the Cross Crawl, the Zip Up, and the Hook Up—are an easy and quick way to wake up your energy, get it moving in the right direction, and remind it to stay there. Doing all four techniques in sequence should take no more than two minutes. If you aren't going to do a physical yoga practice, but are planning to sit in meditation, you can still use them beforehand. Even if you aren't going to do anything but hurry out the door to work, do these on your way to the shower.

THE FOUR THUMPS

Every cell in your body vibrates. There is a pulse and a rhythm to every cell and system of your body. You're already familiar with the pulse in your veins, controlled by the heart, but that is only one pulse in the body. Your breath pulses with its in-out flow. The valves in your body pulse open and closed. One simple way to communicate with your body is to talk to it with pulsation, and you do that by thumping (or tapping) on specific points on the body.

The Four Thumps practice puts this language of body to good use. Put the tips of your first two fingers and thumb together to form a three-point notch. You'll be tapping or thumping that three-point notch against several key points on your body in turn, using a strong and solid pressure, as if you were knocking on a door.

Thump one. The first thump is on a pair of meridian points known as K-27, which are the end points of the kidney meridian. They are located in the slight hollows underneath the end points of the collarbones. Find the round, bony end points of your collarbones with your fingers. Then come down off the end of the bone about an inch into the hollow right beneath. Some people will move their fingers slightly out about a half inch. If you press in and the points feel sore, you've found them! Thump or massage these points vigorously.

All the yin meridians pass through K-27 and then flip over to their corresponding yang meridians, so stimulating or awakening these points has the effect of waking up the entire meridian system and getting the energy in it moving forward. The kidney meridian is considered to carry the earth's vital life force energy (called *prana* in yoga and *chi* in TCM), so working these points also helps to increase and distribute the life chi. This action has its roots in our ancestors, the apes, when they would bang their chests. They are waking up their meridian system and preparing for the day.

For many people, these points are sore. Generally, sore points on the body indicate where energy is stuck, frozen, or compromised, and massaging or thumping these places will help break up the energy and move it. Just don't thump on a point if there is a bruise or injury at the site, or if there is some underlying issue that might be causing the discomfort.

Thump two. The second thump is in the center of the sternum, at the thymus gland. Again, thump or massage this point strongly.

The thymus gland supports your immune system and helps to generate and educate T cells, which helps your body fight disease and correctly identify invaders. The thymus also stimulates all your energies, increasing strength and vitality. This is a particularly good point to work if you feel an illness coming on.

Thump three. The third thump is the end points of the spleen meridian, located on the side seams of your body out from the crease underneath your breasts.

The spleen meridian is responsible for metabolizing food, experiences, thoughts, and energy. If you've eaten a meal that might not have been the best thing for you, thumping or massaging these spleen points will help enormously. If you've had a challenging experience with a friend or a coworker, massaging these points can help you digest that experience. The spleen meridian is also part of the immune system.

The meridian carries the spleen energy of metabolizing (the transformation and transportation of substances) to all the other organs of the body. The physical spleen is also part of the immune system and the blood production and storage systems. It is not considered a vital organ in Western medicine, but the meridian of the spleen (which still exists even if the organ does not) is one of the most important and crucial meridian lines in the body.

There is a second set of spleen points, called the spleen neurolymphatic points, that are located along the same axis as the meridian points, but closer to the center of the body; thumping or massaging these points is also quite beneficial. I tell my students to massage or thump the whole triangular-shaped rib-cage area below the breasts; you're sure to hit the spleen points. And when you find a sore spot, work it!

Thump four. The fourth thump is on the beginning points of the stomach meridian. They are located on the bone directly under the eye, in line with the iris when the eye is looking forward. This delicate bone requires a lighter tap. Use the first three fingers of each hand sequentially to lightly drum on the bone, as if you're drumming your fingers on a table.

Governed by the earth element, the stomach meridian helps to ground your energy. After waking up and activating the meridian energies with the other three thumps, grounding and stabilizing them with the stomach thump is helpful. Tapping these points also helps us to separate ourselves from a problem by enabling us see the difference between the issue and our reaction to it. (You'll begin to see how the meridians have a physical component as well as an emotional component in week 5, when you work with the five elements.)

You can also lightly drum the entire orbital bone that circles the eye. The beginning or end points for three other meridians (gallbladder, triple warmer, and bladder) lie around the eyes, and tapping on the entire orbital bone helps to wake up and energize those meridians as well.

See figure 1 for a complete map of the points to tap for the Four Thumps.

THE CROSS CRAWL

The second portion of the Wake Up will get your energies crossing over throughout your body. Every part of your body contains crossover patterns, from the

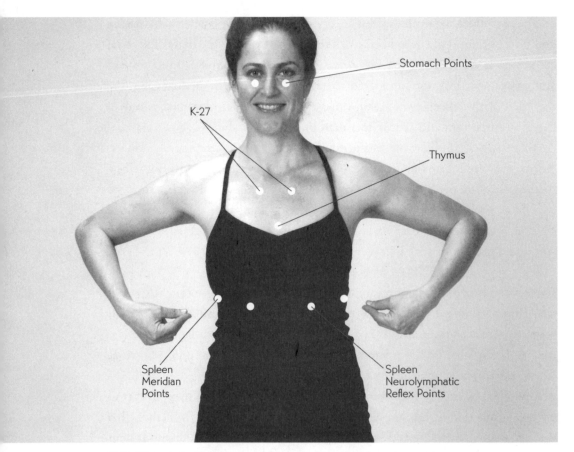

FIGURE 1   In the Four Thumps, we tap on four key sets of meridian points.

twisting ladders of DNA embedded in each cell to the two hemispheres of the brain controlling the opposite sides of the body. Through these patterns, your body communicates and carries out its most integrated functions. These crossover patterns help the body to coordinate its many disparate activities and keep all the energy systems working well together. If the energies of the body are not crossing over, your body is at a deficit and has to work harder to execute its actions.

When the body is tired, run down, depressed, or ill, it will start to conserve energy by shifting its natural crossover patterns into homolateral patterns, in which the energies run parallel to each other instead of crossing over. This switch tells the body to slow down and rest. But sometimes our bodies get locked into this pattern of tiredness. If you have trouble getting well from an illness, are always tired, are more tired than energized after you exercise, are chronically depressed, or simply feel off, it is likely that your energies are running homolaterally. One excellent way to correct this homolateral pattern is to do the Cross Crawl.

Start by marching in place, lifting the same arm to the same leg ten to twelve times. The right hand strikes the right knee as the knee rises; the left hand strikes the left knee.

After a total of ten to twelve of these, brush your hands together as if dusting them off. This momentary break in momentum tricks the energies into taking a pause. Then, when you change your movement to a crossover march, the energies will follow you.

Now do twelve crossover marches in place, with each hand slapping the opposite knee (figure 2). The right hand slaps the left knee; the left hand slaps the right knee. If you find the crossover march challenging, it is quite likely that you need to do it more.

You can do this whole routine three times at a go. Eventually your body will begin to respond to the crossover pattern, but depending on your level of energy, it may take a while. If you are physically unable to do the crossover march standing, you can do the whole routine sitting in a chair, moving just your arms and not lifting the legs and knees at all.

Tip: When I'm hiking in the woods, I often find myself dragging along behind my dog. I'll thump K-27 and then do a Cross Crawl, and instantly I've got the pep to keep up with him. The more you experiment with these Wake Up techniques and use them throughout your day, the more you'll find yourself beginning to understand how your body's unique energies work and how to feed and care for them so they work better.

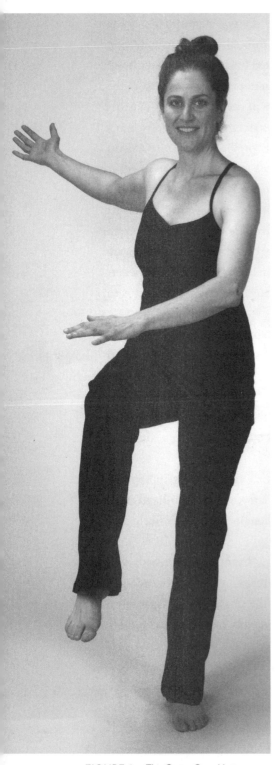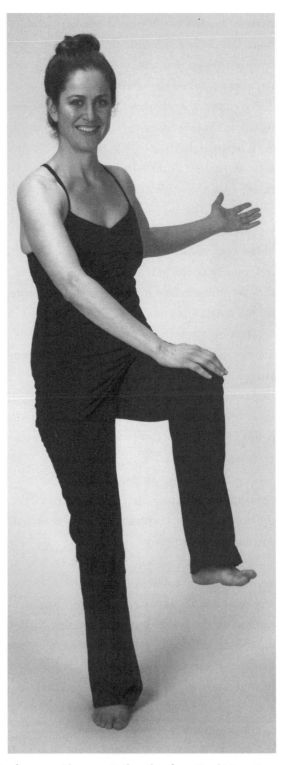

FIGURE 2   The Cross Crawl brings energies from one side across to the other, for optimal integration.

THE ZIP UP

The Zip Up will protect you from other people's energies and the energies of your environment, as well as clear your own mind. Have you ever had someone look you up and down, making you feel naked and slightly icky? Essentially, what that person has done is draw down your energy, making it flow against its natural upward pattern, and this weakens you. This technique of drawing down a person's core energy was used in battle and is still used today in martial arts to weaken an opponent. The Zip Up reverses that process, drawing your energy upward.

Hold your hand in front of your pubic bone, palm facing your body, and run your hand up the front of your body, to the level of your chin. Your hand can be either touching your body or just off the body an inch or two. Because the body is electromagnetic, your hands carry a charge, and your magnetic hand draws the energy of the central meridian upward. The movement is similar to swiping the screen on any smartphone or tablet device.

Tip: You can also use this motion to seal in an affirmation for yourself or set an intention at the beginning of your Energy Medicine Yoga or regular yoga practice. Simply pause with your hand at your pubic bone, take a moment to connect to your affirmation or intention for the practice, and then zip up the words along with the energy.

THE HOOK UP

The next step of the Wake Up is to connect and stabilize the central meridian, which you've just zipped up, with the governing meridian. These two meridians vertically circle the core of your body, and when hooked up become even more potent.

Hold one finger in your belly button and one finger at your third eye, between your eyebrows. Push both in and pull slightly up. Take three deep breaths, inhaling through the nose, and exhaling through the mouth.

This technique is called the Hook Up. Not only does it link your two core meridians, but it is also the single most important thing you can to do strengthen your aura. (See week 2 for more on the aura and how to keep it strong.) The Hook Up helps to stabilize the core of the body, so anything to do with spinal alignment and emotional alignment is helped by hooking up. This is a technique that we use often throughout the Energy Medicine Yoga sequences.

Optional Wake Up Practices: Head Massage, Crown Pull, and Spinal Flush

The next sequence of techniques clears unwanted energies and removes toxins from the whole body. This piece can be added into the Wake Up when you have more time. It is a powerful tool for resetting the whole body and helping to hold off a cold or illness. In week 8, you'll learn another technique for working with the head, utilizing the power of the neurovasculars. The Head Massage and Crown Pull serve as a mini introduction to that technique.

HEAD MASSAGE

First, let down your hair. If you've got a ponytail or clips or pins in your hair, take them out and set them aside. Now massage all over your head, as if you're shampooing your hair. Our heads are covered in neurovascular reflex points, and all of the yang meridians—stomach, bladder, triple warmer, small intestine, gallbladder, large intestine—start or end on the head. Yang is the active, outward-moving, intense energy. Everything we do with our senses except for touch—seeing, hearing, tasting, smelling—is active and engaged and based in the head. As well, we are a culture that spends most of our time "in the head." We figure, plan, problem-solve, communicate, and think, think, think. If we don't find a way to release all the energy accumulated in our heads, that energy gets stuck there and causes all kinds of tension and stress. No wonder so many of us suffer from headaches.

Massaging the head starts to release this built-up energy. If you feel a sore spot, go to the same place on the opposite side of your scalp and see if that sister spot is also sore. Generally the tension in our heads is balanced and often starts in, or is reflected back by, the corresponding out-of-balance organ. If you hold these twin points and massage them, you'll notice that the pain quickly starts to ease.

Pay particular attention to the temporal bone behind the ear and the occipital ridge, at the base of the head, where the skull connects to the neck. These locations are particularly susceptible to tension, and they are the seats of some powerful energy points. We'll work more with these areas in the coming weeks, but for now, if they're sore, massage 'em more.

CROWN PULL

The plates of the cranium are interconnected by a puzzlelike line of joints. These sutures actually move when manipulated. The following technique, called the Crown Pull, helps to keep the joints between the plates supple and can help with headaches and mental fatigue. It's a great technique to do if you've been studying or reading a lot.

After spending a few minutes on the Head Massage, bring your hands together in front of your forehead, curving the fingers and pressing all of the fingertips into the center of your forehead (figure 3). Press in and then pull your fingers away from each other slightly, about an inch or so. Then continue this same motion—pressing in and pulling apart—up and over your head, along the center line of your skull, all the way over the crown, and down the back of the skull, to where the neck connects to the head.

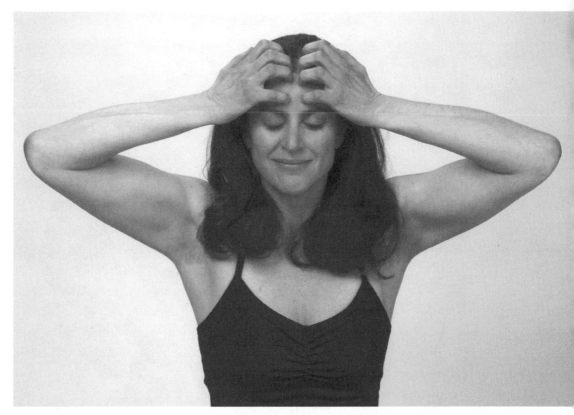

FIGURE 3   The Crown Pull keeps the joints between the cranium plates supple and helps with headaches and mental fatigue.

SPINAL FLUSH

The Spinal Flush is one of the most powerful tools you can use to stay healthy. If you're tired, it can bring you energy. If you're over-energized, it can calm you down. If you're getting sick, it can help keep sickness at bay. In it you'll work the neurolymphatic reflex points, which help flush the entire lymphatic system. And because you're working with points along the spine, the Spinal Flush also helps to stimulate the cerebrospinal fluid.

At the end of the Crown Pull, your fingertips will be at the top of the neck. From here, bring your fingers and thumb back into the three-finger notch (the same finger position used in the Four Thumps) and massage deeply on either side of the spinal cord at the neck; these are kidney neurolymphatic points. Keep massaging down the upper back, on either side of the spine, as far as you can reach. Then pull your fingers, with pressure, over your shoulders. Stop at your shoulders and squeeze deeply; these are the triple warmer release points.

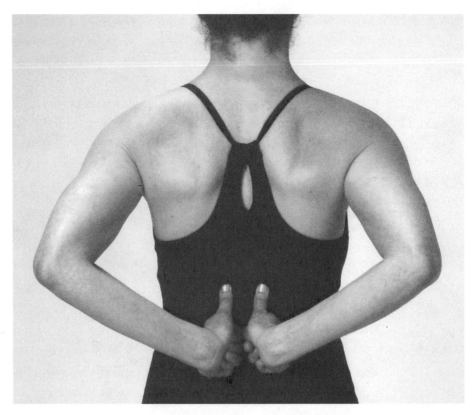

FIGURE 4   For the Spinal Flush, reach as far up the back as possible and massage downward along both sides of the spine.

Bring your hands around to K-27. From here, continue massaging down either side of your sternum. (The neurolymphatic points mirror through the body, so working the points in the front stimulates the same reflexes that the anterior points do.) Continue massaging downward until you get to the point where your ribs connect to the diaphragm, in the center at the xiphoid process, and then drag your hands back around to your back again. Reach your thumbs up as high as you can along your spine and deeply massage down along either side of the spine, all the way to the coccyx. Then press deeply into the center of the butt cheeks, which hold points for the circulation-sex meridian. Pressing here also helps relax the hips and open up the chakra system.

When you're finished, bring your hands up your back again, as far as you can, and sweep them down and off your back three times, helping to clear the energy you've just released.

Tip: Donna Eden recommends doing a Spinal Flush with your partner as a way to release pent-up stress and head off potentially explosive situations, as well as a way to lovingly care for one another. Have your partner sit straddling a chair, with her head resting in her hands on the chair back, or have her lean up against a wall, as if she's being frisked. Work down the back, pushing your fingers or thumbs into either side of the spinal column, with deep pressure. (You'll be working only down the back when working on your partner.) If there is a point that feels sore, spend a bit more time massaging that spot to clear it. Work the points down the spine two or three times, and end by sweeping your hands down the back three times.

More Practices of the Week: Squat and Hang

I start every personal yoga practice with a squat and a hang. These are power poses—essential poses to do even if you're not going to do anything else; they are the poses that give you the most bang for your buck.

One of the predictors of longevity is how easy it is to sit down on the ground and stand up again without assistance. The squat and hang poses are ways to practice these important physical movements.

Many yoga poses are simply variations on the squat or the hang. The squat is a compression, and the hang is an extension. They are yin and yang movements that complement each other.

WHY SQUAT?

Women, men, and children in non-Western cultures spend most of their work and leisure time squatting; they squat as they're cooking, cleaning, shelling peas, sharpening knives, carving wood, smoking pipes, playing games. This position is beneficial in many ways. It compresses the internal organs, helping to move blood and lymph and, with them, toxins and other "used material" out of the organs into the venous blood system for excretion from the body.

This position also helps us keep a deep and fluid flexibility in the hip joints, which is something we all have at birth but which diminishes with lack of use as we age. The hip joints have been called the holders of emotions, and they are also where sexual energy resides—as well as one of the main places where the energy of sexual trauma often gets stuck. A hip joint that is flexible is able to move easily and release emotions instead of keeping them locked into unbeneficial energetic patterns within the body. Also, having supple hip joints is crucial to the proper alignment of the body when we are walking and standing. In our culture we spend far too much time sitting in chairs or in cars and leaning forward, either over a computer screen or a steering wheel or for other types of work. These postures shorten and tighten muscles in our legs (the hamstrings and Achilles tendons) and in our shoulders, necks, and backs. The tendency for the upper back and neck to be out of alignment can be directly related to headaches, rapid aging, and bone deterioration.

Our internal organs need room to move and breathe, and how young our bodies stay, especially internally, can be directly related to the mobility and motility of our organs—the ability of the organs to move easily, bending and compressing as we move, and to have a healthy fluid flow within and around themselves, which helps our organs retain their elasticity. The squatting position helps to reinforce the inherent mobility and motility of organs.

The squat is also the preferred position for childbirth, because gravity and the physiology of the body help the mother push the child out of the birth canal.

Perhaps the most important reason this posture is so beneficial is that it helps with elimination. In our Western culture, where our diets are heavy in processed food, caffeine, alcohol, and other stimulants and depressants, elimination is a universal challenge. People's elimination issues can run the gamut, from extreme constipation to extreme diarrhea. Crohn's disease, excess weight, hemorrhoids, and edema are frequent complaints.

The current use of a toilet that puts the thighs at a 90-degree angle from the hips can be traced back to the royalty of the Victorian Age (hence, its nickname "the throne"). The royals did not want to appear to be close to the earth or close to the peasantry, who would squat to defecate into holes bored in the ground. But the organs of elimination work best when in a squat, which allows the rectum muscles to relax and come into alignment for release. The squat also opens the buttocks away from each other, creating a clear pathway and a more correct opening of the anus for elimination.

A sitting position actually puts a bend in the rectum muscle, which allows us to hold our feces in, helping us to maintain continence. This position is not biologically optimal for elimination.

There are many apparatuses that are intended to help the human body achieve the squat position in the modern household bathroom. There are footstools that raise the thighs to a more appropriate angle, and there are even devices that sit on top of the toilet seat and provide a platform you can use to squat on the seat itself.

All of this is a long-winded way of explaining why we should "reclaim our squatter's rights," as a yoga teacher of mine in Los Angeles used to put it. The squatting pose is one of the most profound, most beneficial poses that you can master and one of the most powerful for keeping the body young.

WHY HANG?

The hang is about lengthening and loosening the back of the body, the hamstrings especially, but also the often-tight low back muscles and shoulder girdle. Hanging over is also an inversion and starts to get the body used to being turned upside down, something most of us stop doing after we pass cartwheel age. Allowing the body to extend this way takes pressure off the vertebrae and allows the spine to lengthen without compression. This also gets us ready for back-bending poses, where we are lengthening the spine, but often also compress it instead of lengthening and opening between the vertebrae. This pose also allows the muscles of the legs and hips to stretch, while at the same time starting to strengthen them. It is also calming to the nervous system. In succession with the squat, it helps to free the hips, calm the mind, and strengthen the lower body.

The following squat and hang poses are ideally done together, but they can also be done separately. In my more advanced classes, I'll go back and forth between the squat and the hang several times, holding each pose for one to three minutes.

These instructions assume you'll be doing the squat first, then the hang immediately after—a two-pose Energy Medicine Yoga power sequence.

SQUAT WITH GAIT CLEARING

Coming into the pose. Spread your feet as far apart as you like, or keep them close together—whatever is most comfortable for your physiology. (If you have large breasts, it might not be easy to keep your feet close together.) You can have your feet parallel or slightly turned outward. Ideally, you want to have the weight balanced on the feet, both back to front on each foot, so that there is a nice lift in the arches, and equally balanced between both feet together. Make sure that your feet are not pronating or supinating—that you are not rolling onto the inside or outside edge of the foot.

If you have very tight hips and hamstrings, you may find that it will take some practice before you can come fully down into a squat. Putting a rolled-up yoga mat or towel into the crease behind your knees and squatting into it as deeply as you can starts to help open up the knees in a safe way. You can also support yourself with bolsters, blocks, and even by holding onto the wall or a chair. For many of us, coming into a deep squat may take time and practice.

Wherever your feet are, make sure your heels are anchored. Place as much padding under your heels as you need in order to allow yourself to "stand" steadily on your feet. Putting a rolled-up blanket under your heels is a good option. Anchoring the heels will allow you to focus the stretch more in the hip region than on the Achilles tendons, which can be very tight. It also helps stabilize you, allowing you to remain in the pose for a longer time. (After you get more comfortable and stable in the pose, you can remove the padding and allow the heels to float as you squat. This version with the heels unanchored will put the stretch and focus more into the ankles and Achilles, while still opening the hips and massaging the internal organs.)

If you still feel unsteady, even with the padding under your heels, feel free to put your hands on the floor in front of you for support.

Once you have come to a squat in which you feel stable, start to deepen your breath. Breathing deeply may seem challenging in this intensely folded position, but that is part of the benefit of the pose. The squat is a type of forward bend, and taking deep breaths while in a forward bend helps to flush out the organs and expand them beyond their usual prescribed place in the body.

I am a big fan of holding poses for a long time, especially in positions such as this, where you can achieve stability without intense muscling. I like to hold this squat for three minutes or even longer. When you start to stretch a muscle, at first it actually goes into contraction out of a reflexive protective response. It takes forty-five seconds to a minute for the muscle to realize it is safe and begin to relax and open up. (Staying in poses for a long time so that deep flexibility can occur is the premise behind yin yoga.) This concept goes perfectly with the amount of time needed to synch up the meridian pulses in the acupressure poses, which we do in week 4. It is also the way to increase your flexibility.

I encourage you to begin to use this pose throughout the day. Perhaps read the newspaper while squatting like this, or do a crossword, or even check your email or your iPhone. I remember being on a boat in New Zealand, and in the front of the boat a group of Japanese tourists squatted as they played cards, drank beer, shelled pistachio nuts, and smoked cigarettes. They sat around in a loose circle, all of them in a deep, easy squat—for *hours!* When they stood up, hours later, they didn't shake out or creak around and swing their legs back and forth to alleviate aches. Instead, still squatting, they gathered all their belongings, then stood up, shouldered their backpacks, and walked off the boat, moving easily, lightly, and gracefully. I can't think of a more healthful posture to use when traveling.

(If you have knee issues or strains, you can do this pose lying down on your back by pulling your knees into your chest. Hug the knees into the body, either one at a time or both together. You'll feel a deep compression in the groins. Try to soften those muscles as you hold the knees into your chest. You can do this pose often, until you feel able to squat on your feet.)

Clearing the gaits. There are five meridians that start or end on the toes: the bladder (on the pinky toe), gallbladder (on the fourth toe), stomach (on the second toe), liver (on the inside of the big toe), and spleen (on the outside of the big toe). Energy has a tendency to get stuck and trapped at these junction points, or gaits. This pose gives you a perfect opportunity to clear them.

Starting an inch or so back from your toes, massage down the tendons between your metatarsal bones. Smooth down into the gullies between your toes and press the skin into the ground as you finish. If you can lift your toes up while maintaining the squat, massage on both sides of the feet by reaching under the toes with your fingers and pinching off at the gullies (figure 5).

You can also clear the toe gaits in the hang, and after a while you'll figure out which position you prefer for this clearing.

Coming out of the pose. Until your body becomes used to this pose, it might feel less than comfortable—not a place where you'd be willing to play a long hand of gin rummy. So coming out of the pose requires using the intelligence you're beginning to develop as you learn to speak your body's language.

Remove the padding from beneath your heels. Then, turning your feet to parallel, begin to lift your buttocks up to the sky. Keep the head hanging down, releasing any tension in the neck and shoulders. Extend the legs straight, but keep a slight bend in the knee. You are now in the hang, the second of our two power poses.

HANG WITH GAIT CLEARING AND INTESTINE DETOX MASSAGE

This version of the hang isn't meant to stretch the hamstrings, but to release the hips and knees, release the compression in the belly region, and release any tension that may exist in the neck, shoulders, and upper arms.

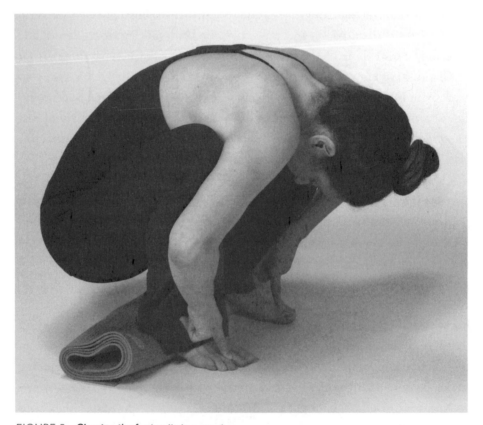

FIGURE 5   Clearing the foot gaits in a squat

While in the pose. As you're hanging over, gently shake the head back and forth, in yes and no motions, a few times. Make sure the jaw and tongue are relaxed. Let the arms hang down. If this feels uncomfortable, hook each hand in the opposite elbow crease and let the whole shoulder girdle release off the spine. It may help to deepen the bend in the knee and then straighten it a few times.

I encourage you to hold the hang for at least a minute. As you feel comfortable after that, you can begin to straighten the knees more, always keeping at least a microbend to accommodate the tendency, especially in women, to hyperextend. With a bit of a straighter knee, you can start to open up the hamstrings, saying a gentle good morning to this perennially tight muscle.

Clearing the gaits. This is the perfect time to clear the energy gaits on the hands. Six meridians start or end in the fingers: the small intestine (outside of the pinky); the heart (inside of the pinky); the triple warmer (ring finger); circulation-sex, also known as the pericardium (middle finger); large intestine (index finger); and lung (thumb). Between the fingers are common places for energy to catch or pool. We are also constantly using our hands, which can constrict the flow of energy there.

Take the right hand and, using your thumb and first two fingers of your left hand, massage down between the metacarpal bones of each of the fingers and pinch off the flesh at the end of each gully. Spend a little extra time on the fleshy bit between the thumb and index finger. You can also massage down the length of each finger, pulling the extra energy off the ends. Change hands and clear the gaits of the opposite hand. (Some people find it easier to clear the toe gaits in the hang and the hand gaits in the squat. Experiment to see which you prefer.)

At this point, take note of how far over you are bent—not with any ego intention, but just to note where your body is comfortably resting. Again, make sure you always have a slight microbend in the knees.

You can slowly stand up to do this next piece, the intestine detox massage, or stay hanging over. If you stand up, do so slowly. Some people find it easier to come out of the hang for this next part, especially the first time they do it. After that, it is easy to do while hanging over.

Intestine detox massage. Take your first two fingers and your thumb, again in the three-finger notch, and massage, with some vigor and pressure, the outside pinstripe edge of your thigh, as well as the inside center line of your thigh, right

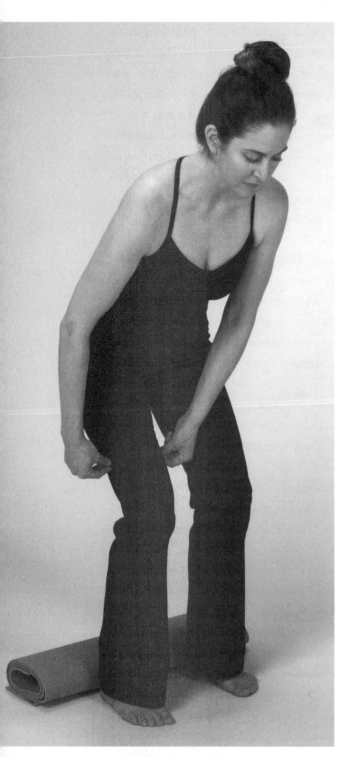

FIGURE 6   Clearing the large- and small-intestine meridians

up to your pubic bone (figure 6). You can do one leg at a time, pressing on both the outside and inside points together. If you are not feeling any soreness or pain, likely you aren't working deeply enough.

This is a detoxification technique, so it doesn't necessarily feel good, but the benefits are huge. If you are prone to loose stools or diarrhea, massage up from the knee to the hip. If you are prone to constipation, massage downward, from the hip to the knee. Use real and significant pressure; don't be meek with yourself! If any points along these leg seams are sore, as they are on most people, you need this massage.

You're working the large intestine and small intestine neurolymphatic reflex points (as well as some circulation-sex points). You are stimulating the lymph from these organs to dump their toxins into the venous blood supply. The intestines are the organs of digestion and waste removal. On a mental level, both the organs and their meridians correspond to the decision-making process and letting go. The body decides what nutrients it wants to keep and what is waste. That chocolate chip cookie you ate last week or that double bacon cheeseburger you ate last month is the soreness you're feeling—the toxic residue of unnecessary or unusable material. That soreness could also be related to that disagreement you had at work that you just can't seem to let go of.

The large intestine contains more neuropeptides in the body than all the other organs combined. It is often called the second brain, because it has more emotional impact on who we are than the brain in our head. The gut creates hormones, including 95 percent of the serotonin in the body, which regulates sleep and lifts the mood. There are also many stress-reducing hormones created in the gut in direct response to the fight-or-flight response. Yet another reason to work these points frequently and keep the intestines healthy.

After you finish your massage, release back into the hang if you had come out of it, and notice if you are able to hang over deeper in the pose. The reason for this deepening is that you've just broken up and moved lymph out of the large and small intestines, located in the low belly, creating more room for the body to fold into.

Coming out of the pose. When you're ready to come up out of the pose, do so slowly. Bend the knees a bit deeper and begin to roll up, one vertebra at a time, until you are standing. Take a few deep breaths to adjust. You are now standing in mountain pose (*tadasana*), and ready for the next part of your practice. If you're not doing any more yoga, you can come from the hang, back into the squat, and then lie down on the floor and rest in corpse pose (*savasana*) for a few moments before continuing on with your day.

Doing the Wake Up plus the squat and hang makes for a powerful combination on its own, as well as a great opening for a longer Energy Medicine Yoga practice.

Sun Salutations and Figure Eights

This week you essentially shake out the sheet of your body to get rid of excess energy and bring the energetic body back to a neutral state. You then guide the energy in the most beneficial directions to help support you.

Energy Systems of the Week: The Radiant Circuits, the Aura, and the Celtic Weave

This week's practices give you a chance to play with three more energy systems: the radiant circuits, the aura, and the Celtic weave. They also support and make use of the meridians, which you've already gotten to know in week 1.

THE RADIANT CIRCUITS

The radiant circuit system is the first energy system that is evident in a fetus. In TCM, the first eight divisions of the fetal cell are actually the eight radiant circuit paths. The radiant circuits are the energies of joy. They resonate with the second chakra, with the innocence, creativity, and vitality of childlike wonder. These energies flow along specific pathways, the same way energy flows through the meridians, but when the radiant circuits are activated, they jump off their paths and fly around freely and exuberantly, going wherever they are needed in the body. I think of them like Tinker Bell, flying around and distributing her fairy dust.

We heal our bodies through the energy of the radiant circuits, because they distribute life force energy, bringing it wherever in the body it is needed. They revitalize the whole body and being and penetrate deep into the cells to facilitate healing and growth. They also store excess energy until we need it.

Music, singing, dancing, and making love are all activities that engage radiant circuit energy. These energies are also highly responsive to thoughts. When that someone special walks into the room and you feel yourself light up, this is radiant circuit energy at play. The fact that just thinking of that someone special makes you feel all tingly is a perfect example of the power of thought to activate the radiant circuits.

Energy Medicine Yoga Sun Salutations help activate the radiant circuits and encourage them to go wherever they're needed in the body.

THE AURA

The aura, also called the biofield, is the protective energetic coating of the body. It can extend from a few inches to several feet off the body. The aura has seven layers surrounding the body, like nesting dolls. These layers, often called auric fields, connect with different energy centers within the body, and each holds different information.

The first layer, closest into the body, is called the etheric field and interacts most closely with the physical body. This layer contains your spiritual essence and body blueprint. It holds the shape and field of information about who you are. The next layer out is the protective layer. This layer folds around and protects the etheric layer and helps protect the body from energetic assaults, including negative energy from other people and environmental interferences. The emotional/mental layer is next, holding thoughts and emotions, images, and your personal reality. The next layer, called the morphic field or habit field, holds the energy patterns of the body, including the five elements (which you'll learn more about in week 5). The next layer is called the celestial layer or the astral body and is connected to the spiritual, guiding forces of your life. Your connection to intuition and divine guidance is held here, as well as your higher purpose. This layer can be accessed through meditation and prayer, as well as through what Ram Dass calls Grace, when peace and joy simply become available to you. The next layer is your life color, consisting of one or two colors that permeate the entire aura and hold the themes of your life. The last and outermost layer is the Celtic weave. The Celtic weave surrounds and connects all the other layers of the aura. It also connects the aura and the cells of the physical body. The Celtic weave is both its own energy system and a layer of the aura, as well as a specific exercise for increasing the strength and vitality of the body's energy systems.

The aura also has seven bands going up and down the core body—one band at the level of each chakra. These bands connect each layer of the aura with each chakra, so the two energy systems can share information.

The entire aura is the body's equivalent of the earth's atmosphere and helps process and digest the external energetic information coming in, including the energy of sunlight and the magnetic field of the earth.

The aura can develop holes or tears for a variety of reasons, including toxins in the environment; using drugs, both prescribed and recreational; and traumatic experiences. These holes or tears can have a significant impact on your health, as they let in energies you want to avoid and allow your personal energies to leak out of your body and energy systems. Illness and disease can be seen in the aura before they manifest in the body, and you can work at an energetic level to stop problems before they manifest on a physical level.

The aura can be seen and photographed, as well as felt. For people who work with energy, this is often one of the first energy systems they can feel with their hands or bodies, or see with their eyes.

Tip: Feeling your aura is simple and an easy way to begin to experience your energy systems as real and tangible. Hold your hands out in front of you, palms facing each other and a few inches apart. Slowly bring your palms toward each other. You may start to feel a slight denseness between them, as if you're pressing against a cloud. This density is your aura. You can also feel other people's auras by slowly moving your hand toward their body. If you don't immediately feel the sensation of density as your hand approaches their body, clear your mind and tune your awareness into your hands.

THE CELTIC WEAVE

All of the figure-eight patterns throughout your aura and your other energy systems together make up what Donna Eden calls the Celtic weave. To her, the pattern of this energy system looks like the Celtic drawing of the infinity sign, with no beginning and no end. The outermost layer of the aura is where the Celtic weave resides. The aura is full of figure-eight patterns, and the more figure eights there are, the stronger your aura is. The energies within the body also move in dynamic figure-eight patterns, carrying information and carrying out energetic functions. The more figure eights there are, the stronger all your energy systems are. There are also other geometric shapes in the Celtic weave, such as diamonds and spirals, but the eights are the most plentiful and powerful.

The Celtic weave connects all of the body's energy systems, knitting them together with a series of large and small figure eights and other geometric patterns. Just as plant stalks are knit tightly together to form a basket, the figure eights in our energy system knit together to form the Celtic weave. The more figure eights there are, the stronger your Celtic weave is. The more figure eights you have in your energy field, the stronger and healthier you are. And the healthier you are, the more figure eights you have.

Eden Energy Medicine teaches about the Tibetan rings, which are powerful figure-eight patterns that cross the body in large patterns on the torso. If you've ever had a shoulder injury, you might have noticed that the opposite hip seems out of whack, too. This is because one of the figure-eight-patterned Tibetan rings is out of balance.

The butterfly bone behind the eyes, the eyes themselves, the breasts, the testes—all these are physical figure-eight shapes in the body. If you simply stand still and make a figure eight with your hips, you start to send a powerful spiral up the core of the body. The sashay walk, which, while generally considered sexy and calling out to the opposite sex, is actually nature's way of sending the figure-eight pattern through the body. Even our blood moves through our body in a figure-eight path. "Wrapped around a cloverleaf of four tough fibrous rings, or cuffs, to which the four heart valves and cardiac muscles are affixed, the heart generates nonstop power by contracting rhythmically . . . over and over . . . without tiring . . . in order to squirt blood along a figure-8 path—first through the lungs to pick up oxygen, then around the body to deliver it," writes Barry Werth in his book *The Architecture and Design of Man and Woman*.

The figure-eight pattern is represented in many different healing traditions. In Western medicine, the caduceus, with its two snakes crossing back and forth, is the symbol of health. This symbol likely came from the yogic tradition of the three main nadis, *Ida, Pingala,* and *Sushumna.* Ida and Pingala cross back and forth over the spinal energy of Sushumna, creating a chakra each time they all cross each other. Together they draw the picture of energetic enlightenment, energy moving upward to the crown.

By drawing figure-eight patterns with and around your body, you strengthen the Celtic weave, which also helps to strengthen each individual energy system and the communication between them all. The arm swings in Energy Medicine Yoga sun salutations are another way to strengthen this pattern, as well as strengthen the aura.

Other Important Concepts: The Vayus

From the tantra tradition of yoga we learn the *vayus,* or "winds," which are the energy flows or the forces of energy in the body.

Yoga teacher Bruce Bowditch interprets the writings of Swami Niranjanananda Saraswati and tells us, "Though the vayus function in unison together, each governing a specific area of the body, they can be thought of as elemental forces that are not just the physical, but govern emotional qualities and mental energies, fundamental to physical, mental and emotional wellbeing."

These patterns are helpful to know as you start to learn specific energy pathways. Energy moves in the body in many ways and on many paths. It can pulse at a specific point, as well as concentrate there. It can travel on lines and designated paths. It can also move in larger waves or fields. Energy moves from disorganization to organization and back again. As you learn about each energy system, you'll see yet another path or field or dynamic shift along or through which energy moves within us. The vayus are the currents and forces of energy and help to circulate prana in their specific areas.

Udana: Governs the throat. *Udana* is the upward flow of energy. It regulates growth, enthusiasm, and inspiration. It initiates exhalation and governs speech and sound.

Apana: Governs the pelvic floor. *Apana* circulates energy from the pelvis downward to the feet. It regulates elimination—both mental and physical—and the processes of surrender and forgiveness.

Samana: Governs the navel center. *Samana* circulates energy in the abdomen. It is the balancing, equalizing flow of energy. It regulates assimilation and digestion, including how we draw energy from food and wisdom from life. It is the force of bringing energy into substance. Also, on a mental level, it determines how quickly we learn or how often we repeat the same mistakes.

Pran: Governs both the heart and the head. *Pran* is the internalizing and vitalizing force. It is energizing and recharging. It rules the physical heart and inhalation, which brings us life force energy. Pran allows us to take in things related to sensory awareness. (Pran is different from prana, which is considered to be the totality of life force energy from which we can draw pran. Pranayama, the breathing practices, is the science of using pran to transform the body.)

Vyana: Governs the movement of energy throughout the entire body as the distributive flow. *Vyana* integrates all the vayus and governs the circulatory systems both within us and in our circulation in the world. It also balances the sympathetic and parasympathetic nervous systems.

We need to have all the vayus working well and smoothly for energy to be able to move and integrate throughout the body. For example, apana (downward-moving energy) and pran (heart energy moving inward and upward) merge in the abdomen to intensify the proverbial fire in the belly, which burns up toxins and melts our resistance to our forward-moving path.

A well-balanced Energy Medicine Yoga practice will keep these energies moving, and you can encourage one particular vayu if there is a problem in its related area. For example, if you have difficulty with elimination, regulated by apana, you might add more squats to your practice (and also massage the neurolymphatic points on the sides of the thighs). If you have trouble speaking up for yourself, you might add shoulderstand or fish pose to help encourage udana. (See weeks 6 and 7 for Energy Medicine Yoga versions of these poses.)

The vayus are potential movements of energy. They don't exist without our consciously using them. Unlike chakras, auras, and meridians, which we don't generally see but which exist within all of us and also within animals, the vayus are energetic potential. You bring conscious attention to them, starting in the areas where their potential resides, and then you use that conscious attention to move the energy in the direction of the specific vayu you're working with.

One very powerful way we communicate with ourselves is by visualizing. You can bring your attention to the throat, bring your consciousness there, and begin to meditate on the rising feeling of udana. The energy then rises through the throat, activating all the upward-moving forces. To activate apana, bring your attention and consciousness to the base of your spine and start to feel the energy pulsing there. This begins to activate the downward flow of energy. In your mind's eye, see the energy flow happening in the body. That's how visualization works—it's preverbal and subconscious, *under* the conscious mind. We will use visualization constantly in Energy Medicine Yoga. Energy flows where attention goes.

Pranayama: Sama Vritti

Sama vritti in Sanskrit means "equal breath." The goal is to make the length of the inhale equal to the length of the exhale. This practice helps bring disciplined awareness to the breath, as well as conditions the lungs and starts to build their capacity.

To help you learn to equalize your inhale and exhale, put a count to the breath. Slowly and evenly count one, two, three, four as you inhale, and then exhale to the same number of counts, until the inhale and exhale are even. As the breath capacity deepens, the count will naturally get longer; just continue to make both inhale and exhale the same length. This is a powerful breath practice to bring the body into balance, and you'll use it throughout the Energy Medicine Yoga sun salutation.

As you start to move your energy in prescribed ways, linking the breath to movement becomes more important. This balanced breath helps to balance the nervous system and bring more equanimity to your practice. This is the breath that, along with the breath practice you'll learn in week 3, will most help you to focus your practice; to start to tune into that important element of communication, listening; and to calm the mind.

The Power of Visualization

Visualization is one of the most powerful tools we have available to us, and it is important in tantra yoga, energy medicine, and Energy Medicine Yoga. There have been many studies done on visualization and its results. In one study, participants were asked to visualize themselves lifting weights, and they increased their muscle mass. In another, they visualized practicing the piano, and the brain synapses fired in exactly the same way as with the participants who actually played the instrument. One study had participants visualize themselves to orgasm.

Athletes routinely use visualization to help them reach their goals. People who are paralyzed are still able to move energy in their bodies with the power of the mind itself. The placebo effect is another reminder of the power of thought to transcend the physical form. Believing in something really can make it so.

All of this is to say that the mind is more powerful than we usually give it credit for. The mind cannot distinguish between real and remembered experiences, which is the unfortunate basis for much recurring trauma; just the memory of a traumatic event can start the cascade of stress hormones that re-creates the experience in the body. Conversely, we can harness this power to visualize things we do want, such as to corral our energies for our healing and strengthening. Working with the imagination also helps to bring us into the unconscious mind to start to communicate with it. It is here that most of our innate power lies, and so opening these lines of communication between the conscious and unconscious mind is a valuable thing to do.

We'll use visualization to help focus our minds on creating our bodies during Energy Medicine Yoga sun salutations, as well as in the warrior series in week 6.

Sun Salutations and the Lost Art of Yoga

Yoga has been practiced for more than five thousand years, but it only started being practiced widely in the West in 1893, when a Hindu monk, Swami Vivekananda, gave a lecture about yoga in Chicago. Bringing yoga, an esoteric, previously hidden practice, into our egalitarian, materialistic Western world was sure to change it, and change it did. Not all the changes were bad: Yoga used to be taught only to men. The most secret, powerful practices were taught only to the highest castes and the most holy men. Now anyone can learn and practice yoga and benefit from its untold positive effects. Anyone can access the sacred texts from which the practices were derived. But as it has moved farther from its historical, spiritual, and deeply reverential roots, yoga has lost a large degree of the power and insight that came along with the cloistered hierarchy of the practice.

Today yoga can be found everywhere, and it is often taught devoid of any larger context or intentional perspective. You can find naked yoga, hula-hooping yoga, hot yoga, power yoga, acroyoga—the list goes on and on. And even more traditional forms, like Ashtanga and Iyengar yoga, are missing the "magical" component that can help transform practitioners in ways they aren't even aware of. The focus of today's yoga is mainly on alignment; or strength building, flexibility, and power; or rehabilitation. Some powerful, more esoteric yoga practices, like deep meditation and pranayama techniques, are still taught in traditions such as kundalini yoga, ParaYoga (a form of tantra yoga), Jivamukti Yoga, and Viniyoga. But very few people are teaching the connection between intention, spirit, and the magical component. One of the meanings of the word *tantra* is "a class of magical and mystical treatises." When I started to synthesize the tantra tradition, with its heavy emphasis on pranayama, visualization, and transformation, with the Eden Energy Medicine techniques that have those same components, I was amazed at how many crossovers there were. I was amazed again at the transformations I saw happen so quickly and that I could only describe as magical. I realized, then, how much the art of yoga had been lost as it transformed into the yoga commonly practiced today.

The magic of yoga is the ability to transform not only your body, but also your mind and, by extension, your spirit. Many people feel great after a yoga class and think it's because of the endorphins released during a high-energy class. But people doing slow and gentle yoga can experience the same great feelings. Why? Although calming and stabilizing the breath is one big reason yoga has this effect on us, the specific intention behind the movements is what really makes yoga transformative. Many cultures, including Native American, Islamic, and ancient Sumerian cultures, have used movements very similar to some of the yoga movements, for prayer, healing, and, we can only assume, physical wellbeing. There are hieroglyphs depicting some of the oldest physical movements performed by humans that look very similar to yoga poses. In Energy Medicine Yoga, we also use specific movements with a very clear intention, and because of that intention and directed attention, the movements can transform us on every level.

The sun salutation, a ubiquitous part of almost every yoga class, is the primary example of movement connected with intention. In this practice, the hands start in prayer position in front of the heart. While in this position, many teachers and students turn inward for inspiration or set an intention for the class, but after that, the intention is often lost.

When I start to teach sun salutations, I ask my students why we do them at all. The answers vary: to warm up, to bend the body into all the different positions possible, to greet the day, to set an intention, to honor the practice of yoga. Only rarely do students say, "To get the energy flowing." And when they say that, they don't usually understand the deeper, more exact meaning of what they're saying.

I believe sun salutations are designed to get the energy of the body moving in the right direction, in line with the directions the meridians flow. In addition, the salutations' process of moving the hands around the body is meant to strengthen the Celtic weave by weaving figure eights into the energy systems, and to smooth and clear the aura. In short, the sun salutation is an opportunity to organize your energy systems and corral all those energies into working for you—a way for you to "groom the mountain" of your energy. If your energies are moving one way and your body is moving another, you will be putting out a lot of effort and not getting anywhere.

Visualization can help us make better use of the energy-enhancing movements offered in the sun salutations. As you're sweeping your hands overhead, weave your hands back and forth in figure eights and visualize light or energy coming out of your hands. I like to visualize that the light coming from my electromagnetic hands is painting my aura or smoothing out and repairing any holes or tears in it. You're also adding more figure eights to your energy field, which, as noted earlier, strengthens the Celtic weave. When I'm doing a sun salutation, any time I sweep my arms up overhead or bring one arm up in side angle pose, or lift both arms up overhead in low lunge, I use the opportunity to weave my hands back and forth in crossover patterns or to deliberately smooth or make circles in the aura as I move (like washing a window). No movement in the salutation is wasted; everything is purposeful.

In the version of the sun salutation practiced in Ashtanga yoga, you hold onto the toes and lift the back up before you jump back into staff pose (*chaturanga dandasana*). This hold-and-movement activates the radiant circuits, as well as strengthens the links between certain meridian pairs. Having that knowledge as you work brings more intelligence to the practice and deepens your intention. We'll talk about those movements more as we break down the Energy Medicine Yoga sun salutation.

Simply bringing your awareness and attention to what you are actually doing as you move through space can have a powerful impact on your overall wellbeing. In yoga, we do so much spiraling up and down, swinging our arms out and around the body. If you apply intention to what you are doing, you will find that you not only go deeper into the "one-pointed mind" of the yoga practice, but also align and balance your energies on a deeper level. In this way, you can reclaim the lost transformative art of yoga for yourself.

Practice of the Week: Energy Medicine Yoga Sun Salutation (*Surya Namaskar*)

The Energy Medicine Yoga version of the sun salutation incorporates a Celtic weave exercise, meridian tracing, a radiant circuits activation, and visualization. It also incorporates a *mudra,* a yogic hand position that influences your energy flow—in this case, the flow of the triple warmer meridian specifically. Week 4 will explore triple warmer in more detail, but for now it is important to know that one of its main functions is to govern the fight-or-flight response. For this reason, any time you have the chance, you calm or release triple warmer.

Once you've played and experimented with this sun salutation a few times, you'll see how organic it is, and you'll start to figure out which variations work best for you. As with many of the Energy Medicine Yoga techniques, it takes longer to read the directions than to actually do them. I suggest reading through the whole sequence to understand the reasons behind the movements, and then start to experiment.

∞

Tadasana with triple warmer/heart mudra and figure-eight arm flows. Stand with your feet hip width apart, feet parallel. Root down through the outside edges and the balls of the feet. Feel balanced evenly over the front and back of the feet. Align your hips over your knees, shoulders over your hips. Lift the chest slightly without hyper-arching the low back. Keep the chin parallel to the floor.

Inhale, and sweep the arms up overhead. Exhale, and draw the hands down in front of the heart into the triple warmer/heart mudra: Put the palms of the hands together; place the thumbs in the center of the chest, which is the heart center, and the tips of the index fingers in the hollow notch at the base of the throat (figure 7). This position will lift the elbows up and encourage you to lift the heart center instead of caving it inward. Your index fingers are resting in a triple warmer neurovascular point, which helps to calm the triple warmer meridian, taking stress out of the pose, as well as connecting triple warmer to heart energy through the heart chakra, bringing them into communication and balance.

As you inhale, slowly lift the arms up and overhead. As you exhale, stay standing upright and slowly lower the arms down in front of your body, crossing them back and forth in big figure eights. Introduce visualization here: imagine a color or light coming out of your fingertips and painting a safe, healing cocoon around you.

Inhale again, and this time weave your hands back and forth, figure-eighting each arm out to the sides and up overhead. Exhale, and make big figure eights with your hands as you lower them in front of you.

Turn slightly to the right side, inhale, and figure-eight up your side body. Turn to the left side and exhale, weaving your hands back and forth back down to tadasana.

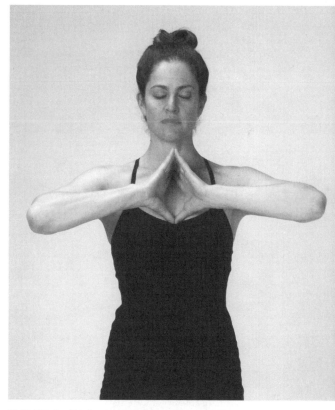

FIGURE 7   Triple warmer/heart mudra connects the heart energy to the triple warmer meridian, to balance and calm this yang meridian.

After several of these figure-eight flows, lower the hands to your sides. Stand still, and see how you feel.

Forward bend (*uttanasana***) with meridian trace.** In order to get a meridian's energy running in the right direction, you want to smooth the energy in the direction the meridian flows. In the next movement, you'll trace the natural up-and-down flows of the yang and yin meridians with your hands as you move into and out of a forward bend.

From tadasana, inhale and bring the arms up overhead. As you start to exhale, cross the right hand over the top of the left hand and smooth the right hand over the outside of the left arm (figure 8). As you get to the elbow, let the left hand come onto the right elbow. Both hands now smooth down the outsides of the upper arms and then down the outsides of your shoulders and upper back, like giving

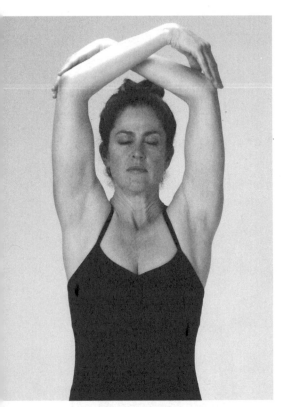

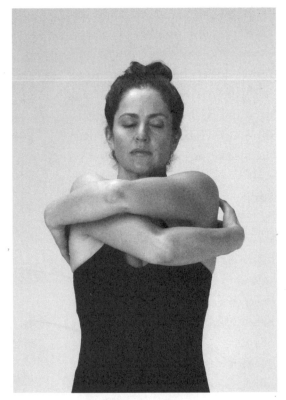

FIGURE 8 Energy Medicine Yoga Sun Salutation: smoothing the yang meridians in their downward directions, a bit awkward over the elbows, helps you learn the contours of the body.

FIGURE 9 Energy Medicine Yoga Sun Salutation: continuing to smooth the yang meridians over the shoulders and the back body.

yourself a hug. This movement may feel awkward, but just allow that awkwardness into the practice, as you're starting to feel the strangeness of the body and its contours. (You aren't folding your torso forward into the forward bend yet.)

Continue smoothing down the outside of the upper back (you'll feel the awkwardness of the elbows crossing again; figure 9) and then pull the hands across the lower rib cage or upper belly, firmly pressing into the belly cavity (figure 10). Bringing your hands around the waist activates the belt flow, a horizontal energy line that divides the upper and lower body at the waist. The only horizontal energy flow in the body, the belt flow is also a radiant circuit, so by tracing it, you are stimulating your joy circuits. The hands cross each other here and then come out to the hips. Start to bend over and continue smoothing both hands down the outsides of the legs, then the outsides of the feet. Sweep the hands off the feet then flick your hands to flick off the excess energy they've accumulated.

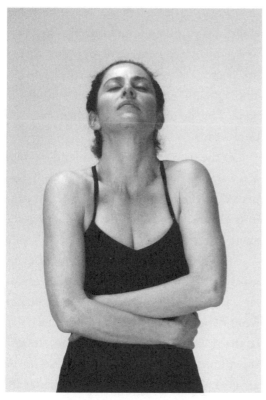

FIGURE 10   Energy Medicine Yoga Sun Salutation: bringing the yang energy across the belt flow, the only horizontal flow of energy in the body.

All of these movements follow the direction of the yang meridians, which run down the outside of the body and into the earth. Yang energies come down from the sun or sky (hence, *sun salutation*). Running your hands over the meridians in this way helps to energize them and get them moving in the right direction, strengthening their flow. The next movement traces the upward direction of the yin meridians, which come up from the earth, helping to strengthen their flow and directionality.

Inhale, and as you start to bring the torso back up, slide the hands along the inside edges of the feet (figure 11), then up the insides of the ankles and thighs, applying some pressure with your fingers. Very often the inner ankles and calves are extremely sore. The more you work these points, the more the soreness will be relieved. When your hands reach the tops of your inner legs, bring them up over the front of the torso all the way up to K-27. Stop here and deeply massage or give a quick buzz, pressing your fingers in and pushing them around at K-27.

Then lift the arms overhead with an inhale. At the top of the inhale and the movement, flick your hands and fingers to flick off the excess energy.

Repeat the entire forward fold with meridian trace again, this time crossing the left hand over the top of the right hand. Again smooth your palms down the arms, over the backs of the shoulders, across the belly. Then fold your torso forward as you smooth your hands down the outsides of the legs. Here, pause, swing the arms forward, and flick energy off the fingers.

Inhale, and again draw the hands up the inside of the feet, ankles, and calves and then up the front of the body. Massage K-27 and then lift the arms overhead. Flick the excess energy off your hands and fingers. Then take one hand, place it over the opposite side of the chest, and smooth up to the shoulder and down the inside of the arm and off the hand. Do the other side, and then shake off both hands.

Do the forward bend with meridian trace a few more times, keeping the breath connected to the movements, and start to tune into the way your hands are shaping the energy over the body.

Tip: When you rise up out of the forward bend and trace up the insides of the legs, instead of bringing your hands up the front of your torso, you can bring them out to the sides of the hips. From there, smooth them up the side seams of your torso to the armpits, and then bring them down again, halfway down the rib cage, and buzz these points. You've just traced the spleen meridian (figure 12). As you'll see in week 4,

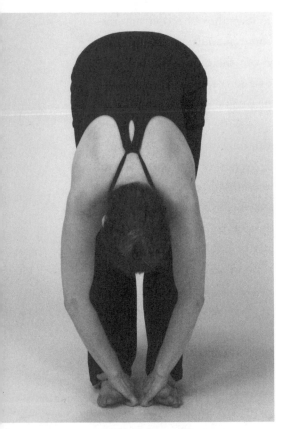

FIGURE 11 Energy Medicine Yoga Sun Salutation: at the bottom of the forward bend, press into K-1 under the foot to start the yin meridian upward flow; this is the point at which earth energy enters the body.

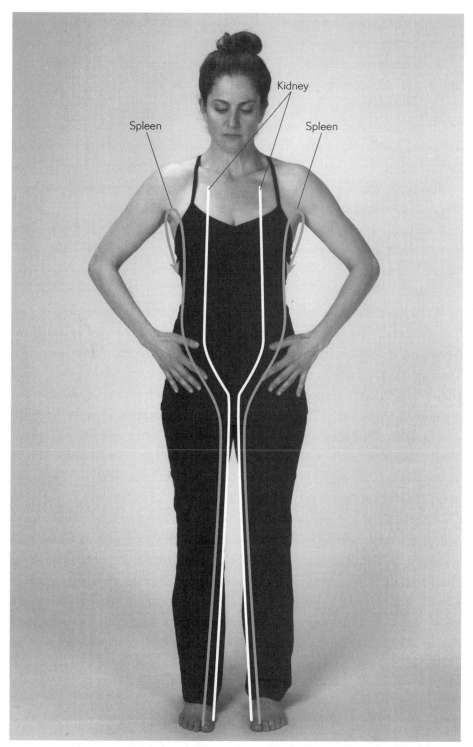

FIGURE 12   Paths of the kidney and spleen meridians, the most important yin-meridian pathways used in the Energy Medicine Yoga Sun Salutation

strengthening the spleen meridian is important for balancing an overactive triple warmer.

We smooth the yin and yang meridians all together, as shown above. The spleen and kidney meridians are so important and powerful that we give their exact pathways here.

Activating the yin bridge flow. Next we'll activate one of the most important radiant circuits, the yin bridge flow. This radiant circuit helps to connect the front and back of the body, as well as balance the yin and yang energies. It also helps to create a bridge between your soul and your higher spirit.

From tadasana, begin by reaching your hands up overhead. Lower them behind your head and press your fingers into the hollow notch at the top of your neck, where your neck and head meet. This is called the power point and is the anchor point for this radiant circuit.

Draw your hands back up over your head and press in at the center of your eyebrows with your fingertips. Draw your fingertips around the inside of the eye at the top of the nose. Then move them under the eye to press in at the center of your cheekbones (the first points on the stomach meridian).

Bring your hands down to your collarbone, crossing them as you do, and press your fingers into K-27. Bring your fingertips together at the heart center, in the center of the chest, and then trace three hearts over your body. Go around the breasts, one hand on each side, then down to the belly button, then up through the center of the body to the thymus again. Draw this body heart two more times. (See figure 13.)

Lastly, fold your torso forward as you draw your hands down the inside of your legs. At the bottom of the forward bend, tuck your hands under the balls of your feet. Pull your torso upward, away from your feet, straightening your back and lifting your butt. With your hands in this position, you are stimulating the K-1 points, the first points of the kidney meridian, located in the center of the ball of each foot. These points are our connection to the powerful earth energy that gives us our vitality and rejuvenation. (This is part of the path of the Ashtanga yoga sun salutation.)

Tadasana with triple warmer/heart mudra. On your next inhale, rise up out of the forward bend, again smoothing your hands up the inner legs and up over the belly and breasts. Buzz K-27, lift the arms overhead, and flick off excess energy. Then exhale and bring your hands in front of your heart, with the thumbs touching the

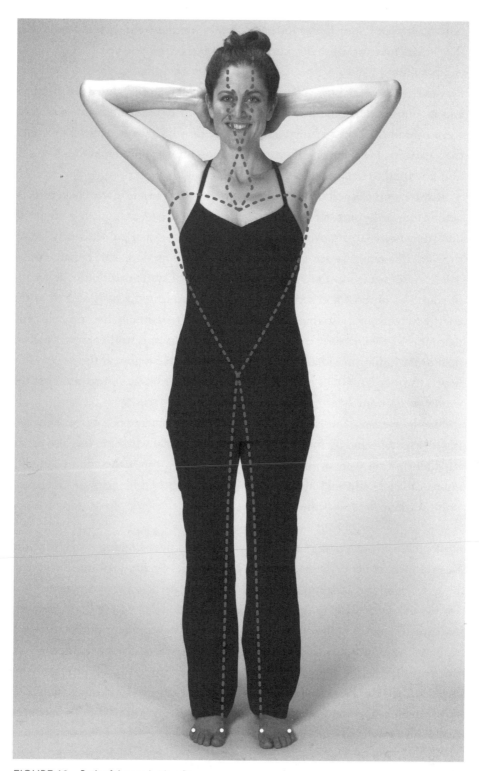

FIGURE 13   **Path of the yin bridge flow**

heart center and your fingertips in the triple warmer neurovascular hollow in the throat. Take three full deep breaths here and center yourself.

Forward bend to chair pose (*utkatasana*) with penetrating flow. Inhale in tadasana, and as you exhale, come into full forward bend. Release the hands and clasp them behind the back, letting your arms fall forward over your head to stretch the shoulders. Hold here and breathe, opening up the shoulder girdle. You may find it helpful to bend the knees a bit.

Release your clasped hands and bring both palms to the lower back, directly behind the belly button. Rub your hands around and around in a circle, in both directions. This movement stimulates the *ming-men* point, which sits on the track of a radiant circuit known as the penetrating flow. This radiant circuit is deeply connected to the health of the hormonal system. It holds the energy of your life's purpose and carries information deep into the body and all of the energy systems. It is also the most spiritual of the radiant circuits and helps you to connect to your sense of self and purpose. Our ancestral energy, which is held in the kidney meridian, unlocks in the penetrating flow. If the penetrating flow is running backward, we get the things we don't want, and we don't get the things we do want.

The ming-men point is one of the most powerful energy points for rejuvenating sexual desire and performance and vitality, especially in men. It is also called the Illumination Gate or the Life Gate; the belly button is the point where life enters the body (through the umbilical cord), and the Life Gate or ming-men point is where life leaves the body.

Chair pose with penetrating flow. Deeply bend the knees, coming into chair pose. Keep the knees bent, the back lifted, and the eyes gazing forward. Finish rubbing circles on the back and pull your hands around the waist to the pubic bone. Stay in chair pose as you draw your hands up the front of the body, between the breasts, and up to the mouth. Cup your hands over your mouth and exhale through the mouth, with a deep sigh, three times. Then fold the hands together, one over the other, on top of the heart center. Stay in chair pose for three more breaths, with the hands over the heart center. This activates your penetrating flow, which is also the main track of life force energy in the body. Chair pose helps you root down into the body as you're drawing this energy up.

To come out of chair pose, inhale, and push the legs straight, to stand. Drop the hands by your sides, close the eyes, and relax into yourself.

Forward bend with meridian trace. Inhale, and come back into chair pose with your hands in triple warmer/heart mudra. Stay for three breaths. Exhale and fold forward, smoothing the hands down the outsides of the legs. At the bottom of the forward bend, reach forward and flick excess energy off the hands.

Chair pose with spleen trace. Bend the knees and lift the torso again into chair pose. As you come up, move your hands from your feet, inside your legs, over your groin, up to the front of the waist and then out to the sides of your waist. Move them up the side seams of the torso to the armpits and back down to the sides of the breasts. Buzz, or quickly massage, this spot. This motion traces the spleen meridian again, something you cannot do too much.

Still in chair pose, bring your hands back into triple warmer/heart mudra and take three to five breaths. Inhale, and straighten your legs to stand. Exhale, and then take a few breaths here in tadasana.

Forward bend with figure eights. Inhale the arms overhead; exhale and move your hands in figure eights as you bring your arms down and fold into forward bend.

Low lunge (alanasana) to extended side angle pose (parsvakonasana). Inhale and step the left foot back, left knee on the floor, coming into low lunge. Make sure the right knee is directly over the ankle. Sink the hips and allow the groin to soften and open. Take three breaths.

Inhale, and slowly lift the right arm up in the air, weaving small figure eights with the hand as you move it upward. Keep the left hand on the floor, creating a gentle spinal twist in your torso. You can extend the right arm forward, over your head, or back down alongside the body.

Experiment with alternately weaving the hand in figure eights and smoothing through your aura in a circular pattern as you move the hand upward. You can also flick each finger with the thumb, both to release excess energy and to wake up the meridian running through each finger. Tapping (or in this case, flicking) the first or last point on a meridian awakens the whole meridian. These movements with the hands and arms are powerful, and as you move through your practice, you can incorporate them anywhere that feels right.

To come into extended side angle pose, exhale and bring the right arm down, balancing the right elbow on the right thigh. Extend the left leg to lift the left knee off the floor, and rotate the left heel down, so that the heel shifts toward the body, and the toes point forward at about a 30-degree angle. See if you can feel the left femur rotating outward as you make this move. You can reach the left arm overhead or keep it on the side body.

Again, use this opportunity to clear the aura, shake off excess meridian energy, and weave in figure eights with your left hand. Take several breaths here, then rotate your body toward the ground and step forward with your back leg. Come down into a supported squat for a breath or two, and then step back the right leg and repeat the sequence on the other side. When you finish the second side, come onto all fours.

Each of these hand and arm moves, and any others you may add, can be infused with the movements of the meridians (as we did coming up and down the body at the start of the sun salutations), the flicking of the fingers (which awakens the meridian energy without directing it), the weaving of figure eights, and the smoothing of the aura. The most important thing is to remain conscious and present, no matter what movements you're making. Continue breathing sama vritti (equal breath), and visualize the beautiful, safe, and empowering cocoon of your energy field surrounding you.

Downward-facing dog (*adho mukha svanasana*) or snake dog variation. From all fours, come into downward-facing dog: Lift the hips up into the air. Keep a slight bend in the knee as you extend the buttocks up toward the sky, lengthening the low back. Feel an outward rotation in the upper arms, embedding the shoulder blades into the back. Don't allow the spine to sink to the floor, hyperextending the back. The goal is lengthening the back, stretching the backs of the legs, and strengthening the core. If your wrists feel sore, try strongly pressing your fingertips into the mat and slightly pulling your body forward, almost like a cat pawing at the ground.

Take three to five breaths and return to your hands and knees.

Many yoga classes stress the alignment of downward dog, using many of the principles I've just shared. I'd like to introduce you to a more dynamic downward dog, one that expresses and engages your unique energies. It comes from Angela Farmer, one of the first senior Iyengar yoga teachers in the United States, who went on to develop her own intuitive style of yoga that includes energy work. She calls this version of downward dog "snake dog," and you might understand why when you try it.

Instead of coming up from all fours into a standard downward dog trying to make sure your alignment is correct, start to breathe into your body and let it move you. Let the energy of your breath and your body, and whatever tightness or constriction you feel, loosen up as you wriggle, wiggle, stretch, articulate, expand, and contract your body. Don't worry about getting into the proper position, but listen to what wants to happen from inside. You might flow into variations of upward dog, three-legged dog, child's pose (*balasana*), side plank, plank, or any combination of poses, or maybe into an unnamable position. Throw out the yoga guidebook and trust your body to open itself up according to its own perfect energy flow. Try shaking yourself and wiggling your spine as you move, and you'll soon see where Farmer found the name "snake dog."

Long-hold plank (*kumbhakasana*). From downward dog, come forward into plank pose, or a push-up position. Make sure your hands are directly under your shoulders. For building strength in the core of the body, including the arms and shoulders, hold plank for up to three minutes. Start building up to this amount of time slowly, adding more time and deep breaths day by day.

Then, start to bend the elbows, keeping them close into the body (not poking outward to the sides, like in a regular push-up), and lower down all the way to the floor. If you can hold the body in a straight plane as you lower, you can pause in staff pose, with your body held a few inches off the floor. Try to hold here for a few breaths. However, if this hold is too challenging, you can lower your knees to the floor first and then slowly lower your upper body, still keeping the elbows tucked into the side body.

Now slowly lower the entire body all the way to the ground.

Cobra pose (*bhujangasana*) with triple warmer rock. With your hands on the floor under your shoulders, lift your head, neck, and shoulders off the floor. Don't put any weight into your hands at first. Press your hips into the floor to extend your low back, and keep your legs and feet on the floor. Engage your stomach muscles by drawing your belly button up toward your spine. It might seem counterintuitive to engage your belly as you're lifting your upper back, but this, in fact, helps to support the low back and prevent it from overstraining. Engaging the stomach also helps to release the tight back muscles and create more flexibility.

Hold your head, neck, and shoulders up for three to five breaths and then release them back down. Lay your hands, one over the other, on the floor in front of your head and lower your forehead onto the back of your hands, completely releasing your neck.

In this position, rock your hips back and forth several times. This sacral rock releases the triple warmer meridian and helps to calm the entire nervous system.

Half locust (*ardha salabasana*) with triple warmer rock. Now lift the left arm and extend it forward. Lift the right leg, and then lift the head and neck. Hold for three breaths and return to the starting position. Rock the hips again. Repeat on the other side, lifting the right arm and left leg. These movements are exactly what a baby does as he is building the neural pathways necessary for moving, establishing the crossover patterns of the body. It is important to release the head onto the hands and rock the hips in between lifts to help calm the nervous system.

Slow cobra with triple warmer rock. Next bring your hands back under your shoulders again. Pressing the hips to the floor, lift the head, neck, and shoulders. After three to five breaths, lower down and turn your head to one side. Keeping the hands where they are, rock the hips back and forth. Turn your head to the other side and rock your hips again.

Now scooch your hands back an inch and slowly start to come up. You'll have more weight in the hands this time, and the work will be slightly lower in the back, maybe between the shoulder blades. Stay here for three breaths, lower down, turn your head to one side, and rock the hips back and forth. Turn your head to the other side and rock the hips again. Now scooch your hands back another inch and slowly start to come up again. You're beginning to see the pattern here.

While slowly creeping the hands back along the side body, you gradually allow the work of the back to shift from the bottom of the neck, where the neck meets the torso, all the way down to the low back. The amount of pressure in your hands increases, while the work of the body is still focused on the back muscles. Make sure you don't feel any strain, and continue to engage your stomach muscles, lifting the stomach away from the floor to stabilize the back. The legs stay on the floor the whole time and as relaxed as they can be. In between slow lifts and three to five breath holds, you'll rock the hips to continually calm triple warmer as you're doing the posture. You'll lift as many times as you want, working the energy down the spine and looking for the most difficult or weakest spot. Once you find it, hold there for an extra breath or two. I usually come up four to five times before I hold at the weakest point and then relax.

When you've completed all of the lifts, bring your hands together, one on top of the other, and let your forehead rest on the back of the hands. This position helps to release excess energy that gets stuck in the head, as well as helps to balance your own energy with the earth energies.

Locust (*salabasana*). Having done half locust pose, you'll now come into the full expression of the locust pose. Lift the head, neck, and shoulders off the floor. Lift the arms as well. The arms can be along the sides of the body, straight out from the shoulders in a T, or in front of you, Superman style. Lift the legs off the floor, too, engaging the low belly as you do. Stay in the lifted position for three to five breaths. When you come down, rest the forehead on the backs of the hands and rock the hips back and forth.

You can do this series of sun salutations, adding any other pieces into it that you like, for as long as you want. When you feel complete, come back to standing in tadasana, or if you're finished with your yoga practice now, bring yourself into savasana and rest for a few minutes, continuing to visualize the energy fields you've just created and cleared.

Working with the Bandhas

Now that you've learned how to move your body's energy along its pathways as well as the flows of the vayus, you'll learn about the bandhas, the locks in the body that help build and contain energy and move it around in larger areas. These work in concert with the vayus as well.

Pranayama: *Ujjayi* (Victory) Breath

The ujjayi or victory breath is the breath used most often in yoga classes. It increases physical power by pressurizing and controlling the breath. It works in conjunction with the uppermost bandha, *jalandhara bandha.* It is also a heating breath and a means of dissipating and controlling pain.

To practice it, slightly constrict the glottis at the back of the throat, forming a whispering sound. Some people call this the Darth Vader breath because of how it sounds. Your breath should be audible to you, but not so loud that someone across the room can hear it. You can do this breath with the mouth open or closed. If you're having difficulty getting the hang of it, put your hand in front of your mouth and exhale a breath into your hand, as if you're fogging a window or a pair of glasses. Then try the fogging exhale again, this time with the mouth closed. You should hear the fogging, Darth Vader sound on both the inhale and exhale.

Ujjayi is powerful to use when practicing poses, but it is not used with other pranayama practices or with meditation, when the focus is on other types of breathing. This is the breath you'll use during most of your Energy Medicine Yoga practice, except during the Wake Up, when you'll breathe in through the nose and out through the mouth. With ujjayi, you're still continually trying to balance the length of inhale with exhale, as done in sama vritti.

Bandhas: Locks for Lifting and Containing Energy

One of the most important ideas related to energy is containment. Think about a garden hose. If there is no attachment on the end and you turn the hose on, the water will simply pour from the open spout, without much force. But if you put a trigger head on the end, the pressure in the hose builds up and can be released in a powerful and directed stream when you pull the trigger. Energy moves and builds up in the body in a similar way, and the bandhas act like the trigger head, helping us to contain the energy and then direct and release it to a specific area with the strength we want.

The bandhas help direct the energy of *agni,* or fire, in the body to help clear blocked energy. The internal fire builds with the directed use of breath, intention, and movement. The word *bandha* means "to tie together, or to close"; it also means "to lock," as in locking in energy. Using the bandhas is a way to lift and hold specific areas of the body so that corresponding energy is contained and moved.

The bandhas are both physical, located as deep in the physical body as we can go, and energetic, responsible for three volumes of energetic space in the core of the body. What is so beautiful about them is they offer a physical way to get into the energetic body.

I've found that T. K. V. Desikachar, in his wonderful book *The Heart of Yoga,* offers the most accessible, easy, and intelligent way to learn and practice the bandhas. He encourages you to find a teacher to guide you, and I encourage that as well. It is always helpful to have someone with experience guide you through new and physiologically different postures. But if you don't have access to a skilled teacher, do not be afraid to experiment on your own. Rely on your inner wisdom (which you are building daily with your personal Energy Medicine Yoga practice) and be modest in your attempts. You wouldn't try to set a bone on your first day of medical school, and yet, if you were presented with a broken bone and there was no one more advanced around to help, you would do your best, intelligently, to attend to the situation.

The first bandha to learn and work with is jalandhara bandha. It is the "net lock" located at the throat. This is the uppermost bandha and allows you to contain energy in the highest point in the body. Because part of the energetics of yoga is to move energy upward from the base of the spine to the crown of the head, it is the most important lock to master. Again, think of the hose: If you do not have a system in place at the top, you will lose all the energy. And conversely, if you have a defective system in place, you could have too much water shooting out of the hose and do damage that way. You wouldn't want to blast a delicate flower with a full-power flow of water, and you wouldn't want to blast your upper-body energy centers with a too-powerful flow of energy.

Jalandhara bandha is the easiest bandha to learn and master. Tilt the chin slightly down, toward the notch in the throat, and pull it slightly back, toward the neck. This position isn't a total compression of the neck, choking off breath and creating a double chin. Think of it instead as holding a ripe peach between your chin and your throat—you don't want to squeeze too hard and squish the soft fruit.

This bandha can be practiced in standing poses and, once you get more comfortable with it, in seated poses.

The next bandha to learn is *uddiyana bandha,* or the "flying-up lock." This bandha is located in the center of the body at the diaphragm, and it is most easily accessed by exhaling all the breath and then drawing the belly button in and up toward the spine. This action helps to lift the diaphragm, which is the goal. Uddiyana bandha is practiced on the exhaled breath. This bandha should not be practiced if you are menstruating or pregnant.

Using uddiyana bandha helps you to bring your awareness and focus to the navel center. If you want to contain and solidify your energy, you must be anchored in the navel. This is the home of the third chakra, which is the center of your ego self, your place in the world, and your feeling of self-empowerment about that place. In order to achieve union with the higher aspects of consciousness (as expressed in the higher chakras of love, communication, intuition, and connection with the divine), you must first have a solid, positive, and grounded place in yourself, which comes from being grounded in the first three chakras (the chakras of home and safety, creativity and sexuality, and personal power, respectively). By anchoring your attention in the third chakra—called the *dan tien* or power center in other traditions—you are able to reach higher levels of consciousness and fulfillment without losing yourself. This awareness in the third chakra is the proverbial fire in the belly. The navel also holds our primordial chi, the original life force energy that animates us. That fire is both the passion you need to do your work in the world, as well as the internal energy you need to help destroy toxins, both physical and mental, that may keep you from fulfilling your potential. Helping destroy internal toxins is one of the purposes of the bandhas.

A tree can only grow as high as its roots go deep, and so deepening your roots and grounding in your lower chakras is important, especially when talking about the flow and power of energy within the body. By using uddiyana bandha to place your awareness and bring physical activity into the abdominal center, you anchor yourself in a very real and primal place. (For more on the chakras, see week 7.)

The third bandha is *mula bandha,* the "root lock." It is located between the anus and the genitals, at the root of the body. The easiest way to begin to feel mula bandha is to practice stopping the flow of urine. Engaging mula bandha feels similar to doing Kegel exercises, which pregnant women are taught to strengthen the muscles of the perineum on the vaginal floor. It is equally power-ful for men, just perhaps not as familiar. Jivamukti Yoga co-founder David Life (one of the most important yoga teachers in the US) once said it is impossible to be depressed if you're using mula bandha, because with it you're directing your energy upward, while depression is a constant downward-moving energy. Mula bandha is the bandha most often used in yoga poses, as it helps to strengthen and stabilize them, and it is the one that you will find most immediately beneficial.

Uddiyana bandha and mula bandha are often linked together; uddiyana bandha holds the upper muscles of the core, and mula bandha holds the lower. They can also be separated and practiced each by themselves.

Mula bandha helps to lift energy upward, uddiyana bandha holds it up, and jalandhara bandha keeps it from exploding out the top. After directing the vayus to help increase agni, the fire energy, to burn through toxins, you then use mula and uddiyana bandhas to lift and hold the fire energy up, and jalandhara bandha to keep a lid on it.

So how do the bandhas actually work after you learn how to activate them? Imagine a balloon filled with sand—a large, oblong balloon, maybe the size of a medium pumpkin. At the bottom there's a tie: the first lock. Halfway up the balloon there's a cinch, like a belt; this is the second lock. At the top, there's a seesaw lever that when pressed down in front lifts up the rubber of the balloon in the back; that's the third lock. When you move these three pieces around, you change how the balloon moves in relation to itself and how it holds its shape. You move the bottom tie to the right and the sand starts to spill over left, so you press one end of the seesaw lever up and displace some of the sand there, and the center realigns and rebalances. The balloon never tips over; it just keeps shifting to stay in balance depending on where those three fulcrum points lie.

The body is not built as a weight-bearing structure like a house. It is built in spirals, and domes, and opposition and tensegrity. Tensegrity means that there is an internal and ever-moving center point that everything lifts around and operates from. There is no downward tension save for gravity. The bones and muscles align and suspend under alternating tension and compression. They don't connect and hang. These are the principles that Buckminster Fuller used to design his domes, the most stable man-made structures there are.

What keeps that tensegrity intact in our bodies is the bandhas. The bandhas are both automatic and moveable, like the breath. However, if we don't move them ourselves, intentionally, by practicing with them, they will cease to work on their own. You can see the results of that in the sagging, downward trends of energy in aging populations.

Working with the bandhas physically helps you to understand how they work energetically. You start to see that the energy body can be a mirror of the physical body.

The best way to familiarize yourself with the bandhas is by standing in tadasana or by lying on your back with your arms outstretched overhead (*tadaka mudra*). In those two postures you can start to engage the bandhas, first one at a time and then in concert with each other. You start to get a feeling for the power and control they offer.

To engage jalandhara bandha, lengthen the spine and tilt the chin slightly down and toward the notch in your throat.

To engage uddiyana bandha, as you exhale, draw the belly button in toward the spine. By the end of the exhale, the belly button and diaphragm should be lifted in and up.

To engage mula bandha, squeeze the muscles at the floor of the perineum, the lowest muscles in the core of the body. This can be done on an inhale or exhale, but as you're starting to learn it, the best way to practice it is on an exhale. Then you can start to see how uddiyana bandha works together with mula bandha on the exhale.

It is a good idea to practice the bandhas one at a time until you feel comfortable and understand their functions. Then you can begin to work with them together.

Slowly you can begin to introduce the bandhas into your yoga practice, making sure that you are not disrupting your focus and breathing by adding too many elements at once. Take one pose once a week, try using one bandha with it, and see how it makes you feel. Once you feel comfortable using the bandhas, you can use them modestly within your practice.

Tip: It is important not to overuse the bandhas. They should not be used throughout your entire yoga or Energy Medicine Yoga practice. They are most useful to help balance and stabilize you in balancing postures and to help focus attention in meditation preparation. They also can help to stabilize and focus the core in strengthening exercises.

SPECIAL NOTE TO WOMEN

Many women learn the Kegel exercises to be used before and after pregnancy to strengthen the perineal floor. Kegels are a good precursor to using and understanding mula bandha. But as a woman, you have an additional tool and center of power that men are lacking.

The vagina, which is actually the entire canal from the exterior opening to the mouth of the cervix, is a muscle that can be strengthened and represents, truly, the innermost core strength of a woman's body. There are many practices that have been used for centuries by women for this exact purpose. In ancient China, such practices were hidden wisdom, used only amongst the empresses. The practices were known to contribute to longevity and strength that went well beyond a woman's physical age.

The Kegel exercises are a way to start utilizing these muscles. If you draw your focus deeply inside your body, you can begin to contract and feel these powerful muscles. The more you practice, the more accessible they will become. Strengthening these muscles not only helps with childbirth and sexual pleasure, but also helps keep the reproductive organs healthy and contributes to the overall vitality of the body. There are references in the back of the book for more information on these esoteric and powerful practices.

Practices of the Week: Working with the Bandhas

The first two poses you'll learn will help you understand and experience the bandhas. There is also a power pose, incorporating more neurolymphatic cleansing in a modified inversion. I also introduce another radiant circuit pose and a way to connect with and calm the nervous system.

CAT POSE (CHAKRAVAKASANA) WITH MULA BANDHA

This pose is a powerful way to experience mula bandha for the first time or deepen your focus on it if you're already familiar with it.

Come onto your hands and knees. Make sure your hands are directly under your shoulders. Spread your fingers out, but don't strain to make them as wide as they can possibly go. Experiment with making a slight claw of your hand, thereby awakening the arches of the hand and allowing the musculature of the entire arm to be engaged. Inhale here.

Exhale and come back into child's pose, with your hips on your heels. Make sure your hips land first, then your elbows, and lastly your head. Inhale, and come back up onto all fours. Do this movement several times, working to equalize and expand the breath and connect the breath smoothly to the movement.

Engage mula bandha on the exhale, drawing the perineum up as you bring your hips back. By exhaling as you sit back, you can really feel the engagement of the bandha, almost as if you're sitting into the bandha itself.

THREAD THE NEEDLE (*SUCIRANDHRASANA*) WITH YANG BRIDGE FLOW

Come into neutral position on all fours. Take the right hand and reach it through the space created by the left knee and the left hand. Draw the arm and shoulder through until the back of the right shoulder is on the ground or close to the ground. Take several breaths here. Deepening your breath in twisting poses such as this one helps to clear toxins.

Now take the left arm and reach it behind the body. Start to draw figure eights on the back as far up and down the spine as you can reach, using either the palm or back of your hand. This activates the yang bridge flow, one of the radiant circuits. It helps to connect the front and back of the body, as well as to bridge the opposites in the body: the polarities, the yin and yang energies, the impulses moving in and out of the body. The yang bridge flow helps us connect to other people as well, to see their true essence and to see them clearly.

Draw several figure eights on your back, then unwind and come back to all fours. Repeat the twist and tracing on the other side. Once you've done both sides, come back to all fours.

Now bring the top of the head to the floor and reach both hands behind your legs to hold onto the back of the knees. Holding the backs of the knees, lean forward, with weight on your head. The backs of the knees hold two of the anchor points for the yang bridge flow, and holding them helps to anchor these energies in the body. This is a variation on rabbit pose (*sasangasana*), with the hold at the knees instead of the feet. If this position feels challenging on your neck or if you have any neck issues, don't do this. You shouldn't have real pressure on your neck, but it may feel awkward if you're not used to putting any weight on the head at all. If you don't want to do this spine lengthening, you can come into child's pose, with your hands pressed to the backs of the knees, compressed by your folded legs.

To come out of either variation of the pose, simply remove your hands from the backs of your knees and come into child's pose.

CHILD'S POSE (BALASANA) WITH SPINAL FLUSH

Child's pose offers a wonderful opportunity to do a variation on the Spinal Flush you learned in week 1. After doing the thread the needle sequence with yang bridge flow and then resting in child's pose, reach your hands up your spine as far up as you can and massage down along either side of the spinal column. This is the path of the bladder meridian, which governs the nervous system. With this massage, you are connecting with and calming the nervous system, as well as clearing lymph and stimulating the spinal muscles.

After working your fingers down along the spine to the coccyx, deeply work the points at the center of each butt cheek—key points of the circulation-sex meridian. Working them helps to calm and open the first chakra, which supports the opening of all the other chakras. Those points also open and calm the energy of the legs. You can finish by massaging the bottoms of the feet, which is the starting point of the kidney meridian, and then squeezing the widest part of the foot, which stimulates the radiant circuits and completes the work on bladder, which ends at the pinky toe.

DYNAMIC BRIDGE POSE (*SETU BANDHA SARVANGASANA*) WITH NEUROLYMPHATIC CLEARING

Bridge pose, a backbend done while lying on your back, is one of the power poses of Energy Medicine Yoga—one of those "more bang for your buck" poses to include in your daily practice or in a short practice when you don't have a lot of time. Bridge strengthens and stabilizes the hips, thighs, and back. It is also an inversion, and helps bring blood flow to the brain and stimulates the thyroid and parathyroid. It is an easily accessible backbend, great for beginners, with many ways to make it more advanced and dynamic. It is also one of the best poses for experimenting with all three of the bandhas.

Begin by lying on your back, arms by your sides. Bend the knees and place your feet flat on the floor, hip width apart. Make sure that your feet are parallel to each other, not duck-toed out or pigeon-toed in.

To begin, inhale and lift the hips off the floor until your body is in a straight line from the hips to the knees. Your body will be at an angle to the floor, but all in one plane, without the hips pressing up above or dropping below the plane of the spine and thighs. Exhale and return the hips to the floor.

Now inhale and lift the hips again and, at the same time, lift the arms overhead onto the floor behind you. This action helps to open up the rib cage, deepening the breath and bringing stabilized mobility to the shoulders. Exhale, returning the hips to the ground and the arms to your sides. Repeat this movement a few more times, then pause and hold at the top of the motion—hips up, arms up.

Inhale and, keeping the hips lifted, lower the arms back down to the sides. Continue to breathe with a smooth, equal breath with the hips still lifted. Release the gluteus (butt) muscles; this will strengthen the back and keep you from jamming the lower back muscles. It may seem challenging to keep your hips up without these large muscles, but what you notice is that almost instantly the work of the pose will go into the low back and the low belly, helping to stabilize the pose. It will also force you to use your feet to really anchor the pose. The weight should be on the shoulders and the feet. This version of the pose will train you to use the smaller muscles along the core of the body, instead of the larger gluteus muscles that we usually default to.

After three or four breaths in this position, lower your body down to the floor. Let your knees fall inward toward each other to release the low back, and take a few breaths. Finish by simply breathing in the pose and releasing excess energy, perhaps with one or two exhales through the mouth.

If you're unfamiliar with the pose, give yourself time to learn it, and then, as you get more comfortable with it, take one to three breaths, practicing each of the bandhas. The neck position naturally engages jalandhara bandha. On an exhale breath, contract the belly button into the spine, engaging uddiyana bandha, and lower down to the floor holding the bandha. When you get to the floor, release the bandha and take an inhale. Try this a couple more times: lift up on an inhale, exhale the breath and engage uddiyana bandha, and then release to the floor. After three of these, do the same practice with mula bandha. After three of those, you can try holding all three bandhas for a moment and then releasing.

Then hold the pose again without engaging the bandhas. Simply breathe there and release the excess energy that will have built up from being contained behind each lock. Take one or two long, slow exhales through the mouth to expel that energy before lowering the hips to the floor.

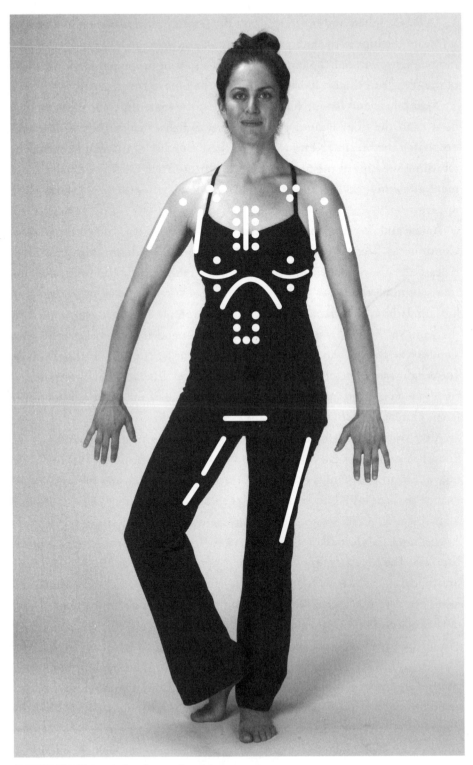

FIGURE 14　The neurolymphatic reflex points

While you're lying on your back, the next part of this pose is to massage the neurolymphatic reflex points along the front and sides of your body. You can refer to figure 14, but these points pretty much cover the trunk of the body and the inner and outer seam on the thighs (you've already worked these thigh points in the hang). Go to where your hands are drawn. If you come to an area that feels particularly sore, spend some extra time there (as long as the soreness isn't due to a bruise or injury). Working the neurolymphatic reflex points helps connect all the meridians together, as well as deeply detoxes the body. Working them at this point in the dynamic bridge pose sequence is powerful, because you'll be lifting up into the inversion one more time, and that will help move the lymph and toxins you're releasing with the massage. You can also try clearing the points while lifted in bridge.

When you've finished working those points, come up again into bridge pose. Again, release the buttocks and use your low back muscles, making sure to stand solidly on your feet so that you aren't crunching up the low back. This time, if it feels right, you can roll your shoulders under your body, bringing your shoulder blades together, and clasp your hands under your back, forming a convex arch with your back. Keep lifting your breastbone up and pressing your hips up as you breathe slowly and deeply for three to five breaths.

When you've finished, come down and breathe. While relaxing for several breaths, continue to work the neurolymphatic points, especially any that were particularly sore. If the points are quite sore, just work a few at a time. If you work too many points too deeply and all at once, you could release a big detox load into the body that may make you feel sick. Be gentle with yourself, even as you're working strongly.

The Triple Warmer and Spleen Meridians

This week you'll discover the power of balancing the triple warmer and spleen meridians, and learn how to work in a more direct way with the meridians to affect the endocrine system and calm the stress response. Having just learned the bandhas, you'll now look at the three locks from the window of the triple warmer energy system, which governs the areas of the body the bandhas control.

Pranayama: The Pure Breath

Rod Stryker calls the pure breath one of the most potent breathing practices for smoothing out long-standing psychological issues. It is also a simple breath to learn, though not so simple to master. This breath helps calm hidden disturbances in the body. Practicing this breath after you've done triple warmer–calming poses can be very helpful.

The breath is a reflection of the emotional body. Conversely, the breath can affect the emotional body. As you've been deepening your breathing practice with sama vritti, you've probably noticed that the breath isn't always smooth. There are gasps, held spots, sharp inhales, blowing exhales. With the pure breath, you start to smooth out these impurities. The goal of this practice is to entirely erase any fluctuations in the breath, including the pause at the top of inhale and the pause at the bottom of exhale.

This practice is best started lying down. When you're more comfortable with it, continue to practice in a seated position.

While lying down, inhale slowly and deeply. You want to create no sound and no wind with the breath. It should be almost invisible. If you notice there are skips or stutters or rough movements, try to ease over them the next time you pass by. When you get to the height of the inhale, you have to deeply relax, especially in the diaphragm in order to turn the breath around without the pause. The same thing goes for the bottom of the exhale. Little by little, you'll shift into a breath that is quite deep, but slow, and has no sound. Breathe as if the breath were one continuous flow. It is no longer inhale, pause, exhale, pause, but one continuous, smooth, pure breath.

I suggest working with this breath several days a week or making a commitment to spend one to three months practicing daily. You can do a short practice with the breath before or after your physical practice. You can also spend some time practicing this pure breath in bed in the morning before you get up, as lying down is the easiest way to start to smooth out the imbalances.

Energy System of the Week: Triple Warmer

The triple warmer is a single meridian, and when positively activated, it can act like a radiant circuit. Because the triple warmer meridian is so strong and plays such a powerful role in the body, Donna Eden categorizes it as its own energy system. "Triple warmer is the meridian that networks the energies of the immune system to counter an invader," she writes in her book *Energy Medicine.* She adds that triple warmer "is governed by the hypothalamus gland, the body's thermostat and the instigator of the fight-or-flight response." Its name comes from the fact that it has three sections—the lower, middle, and upper warmers or burners—each of which occupies and governs a specific area of the body. One of its primary functions is to distribute heat and moisture throughout the body.

The lower warmer is in the low abdomen, the middle warmer is between the chest and the navel, and the upper warmer is in the head, neck, and chest. Triple warmer governs the functions of all the organs, gathering and distributing to the organs energy taken in from food and liquid. It also regulates heat internally and on the skin's surface, keeping the heat balanced or adjusting it to fight or flee a stressful situation. It floods the upper body with heat when preparing us to fight, or floods the legs with heat to prepare us to run. Triple warmer is in communication with every organ and meridian and, therefore, every process of the body. It gathers and disseminates information throughout the body.

The areas of the three burners roughly correlate with the areas controlled by the three bandhas. By learning to use the bandhas with intelligence, you can start to tap into the deeper power of triple warmer. When you start to use the bandhas and triple warmer together—for example, using the triple warmer–calming poses you'll learn in this chapter in addition to the bandhas—you start to gain more access to this energy system, a process that can seem confusing. By utilizing the bandhas, you let triple warmer know that you understand the movement of energy and know how to support the body, so that triple warmer can relax and stop throwing the body into the fight-or-flight response at every loud noise.

The energy of triple warmer is the energy that activates the immune system. As a meridian, the triple warmer is considered to be one half of the immune system and acts as the general in that system. The triple warmer meridian is responsible for the movement and distribution of solids and fluids throughout the body, as well as the movement of energy responsible for regulating all the organs. It also rules and is ruled by the hypothalamus, which governs all the hormonal activity in the body. The triple warmer meridian has the ability to take energy from every other meridian in the body, except the heart meridian. The problem is that triple warmer has not evolved as quickly as the world around us, and as a result, it often overreacts to perceived threats, which then throw our immune system into overdrive.

Allergies are perfect examples of an overactive triple warmer. There is nothing inherently threatening about a peanut, but some people will literally die if they ingest one. This is because triple warmer identifies the allergen as being more dangerous than it is and activates the immune response. In deadly allergy cases, the meridian refuses to see the innocence of the substance and continues to conscript all the energies of the body to essentially fight itself. Immune system diseases like multiple sclerosis and Parkinson's are also examples of the triple warmer meridian gone haywire. Triple warmer identifies the structures and functions of its own body as dangerous and starts up the immune system's fight response.

"The problem solved by the human immune system is the problem of determining 'self' from 'nonself.' This . . . involves sophisticated notions of identity and protection—at cellular and molecular levels," writes Barry Werth in *The Architecture and Design of Man and Woman,* his book with Alexander Tsiaras. But sometimes that system of determination goes haywire and serious problems ensue.

One of the most powerful things Energy Medicine Yoga can do is to calm triple warmer and reeducate it to be more intelligent. We have specific techniques to let it know that the body is safe, that there is nothing dangerous going on, and that it can calm down and support the healthy processes of living. Other techniques use triple warmer to help minimize the impact of stress on the body by calming the stress response in a stress-inducing pose. This allows the body to practice staying calm in the face of challenges.

There are times when strengthening triple warmer is needed, such as during an asthma attack or when someone is going into anaphylactic shock. You can see, by the extremity of those examples, how powerful triple warmer is in keeping us alive.

Triple warmer also governs our habit fields. The reason you can get into a car and drive is because triple warmer holds the habit memory of how to operate a car. But it can also keep you stuck in negative patterns, such as smoking or drinking, even when you want to quit. The energetic habit field is simply too strong; what this means is that the energy of the habit is deeply engrained. The neural pathways in the brain have created a strong connection, and just your deciding to change that connection is not enough to do so. Neuroscience shows us that neurons that fire together, wire together. In the yogic tradition, our habits are governed by our *samskaras,* or the deep imprints in our mind, and our *vasanas,* or our tendencies to make particular choices. Being able to understand and work with these imprints and tendencies can help shift patterns, and utilizing some of the techniques outlined in this book can help you to interrupt and change the flow of these habit patterns. But first, you need to understand how triple warmer operates.

When triple warmer acts as a radiant circuit, it allows you to see your connection with all that is. You are connected to the universe and see your oneness with the world and your own inherent perfection. And that is the goal of the yogic path as well. Triple warmer can help us activate to our higher purpose. Feeling safe makes triple warmer relax. Our *purusha,* or our eternal soul, knows that we are safe, but our earthbound bodies sometimes struggle to remember that. Part of healing this divide is working with triple warmer. When this divide is bridged and triple warmer becomes a radiant circuit, and we have regular access to that feeling of safety, contentment, and oneness with the universe, we have an easier time following our *dharma,* or our life path—an easier time fulfilling our purpose or destiny. We have the clarity to see what needs to be done and the courage to do the work.

The fact that triple warmer does so much and can be so confusing to identify and calm when energy systems go awry is why it qualifies as its own energy system.

Balancing Triple Warmer and the Spleen Meridian

There are many energy medicine techniques that balance the energy of triple warmer with that of the spleen meridian, which is the second meridian that governs the immune system. In Donna Eden's book *Energy Medicine,* she tells us about the importance of the spleen meridian: "Spleen meridian governs the spleen and pancreas, and it is also involved with the thymus, lymph, lymph nodes, tonsils, and bone marrow. It oversees your blood supply, metabolism, homeostasis, the production of antibodies, and the distribution of nourishment throughout your body. . . . Its model of protection is to foster a vital defense by maintaining a vital organism."

The spleen meridian works to keep all of the energy systems strong and healthy. It is considered the most yang of the yin meridians in that it is the most active. Each meridian has a daily two-hour time frame in which it is at its peak or high tide—when its energy is the strongest. For the spleen meridian, that time is 9 to 11 a.m. During this same time period, triple warmer, which sits opposite spleen on this two-hour flow wheel of the meridians, is at its low tide. The tides of these two meridians are reversed twelve hours later: from 9 to 11 p.m., triple warmer is at its peak, and spleen is at its low tide. This relationship means that when triple warmer is weak and needs to take energy from another meridian to strengthen itself, the first meridian it will target is spleen, its opposing energy on the wheel. Since the spleen meridian's job is to make sure all the other meridians and energy systems are doing their jobs, our entire energy system is disrupted when triple warmer steals spleen's energy.

Imagine this: You're feeling ill, and the spleen meridian, being the great mother of the meridians, is corralling its forces to help. Among its tasks are feeding the blood, removing the toxins that are making you sick, and making sure all the other meridians are doing their jobs well. But triple warmer feels threatened by this illness. Because triple warmer is often on high alert, it takes all of spleen's energy for itself and amps the body's response up another notch. So now, instead of being able to heal, your whole body is trying to stop the soldiers from fighting amongst themselves.

Triple warmer often feels threatened and goes into an overactive response, rousing our entire energetic army to get excited about things it really doesn't need to get excited about. A simple thing like hearing a loud noise puts the subconscious at high alert and often compels triple warmer to respond. A fight with your spouse, a piece of bad news, a computer crashing before you've saved the file—all these can trigger triple warmer into action.

On the other hand, if we strengthen the spleen, which in turn helps the other yin forces of the body run well, triple warmer can relax. Triple warmer feels safe and can relax its hypervigilance when the yin meridians, controlled by the spleen meridian and responsible for the lion's share of energy that keeps us alive and functioning, are doing their jobs.

In most people, the spleen meridian's energy is depleted. Especially in our Western culture, where stress is endemic, constantly depleting spleen energy can unbalance the immune system, weaken the hormonal system, and lead to major stress-related and immune-system disorders. For most people, strengthening spleen meridian and calming triple warmer are called for.

When in balance, the triple warmer and spleen meridians work well to protect us. When they're working together, they promote feelings of safety and support our ability to handle the demands of life. They can also literally save us in an emergency. When balanced, this meridian coupling fosters feelings of joy, forgiveness, and gratitude, and inspires warm and balanced social connections.

Because the most powerful meridian dynamic that can negatively affect us is between triple warmer and spleen, balancing the energies of these two meridians is something we'll do often in Energy Medicine Yoga.

Another important reason to strengthen the spleen meridian is that it is one of the two meridians that tend to weaken most as we age (the kidney meridian is the other). "Spleen governs the metabolism . . . how quickly the body can restore and replace natural hormones, the body's ability to renew itself, and the vitality of the sexual organs," Donna Eden writes in *Energy Medicine for Women*. "Strengthening spleen meridian is a way of keeping your entire body strong."

Helping the body stay strong and young is also one of the most frequently given reasons for doing yoga. There are practices described in the Hatha Yoga Pradipika (one of the oldest and most revered yoga texts) that say you will retain the body of a sixteen-year-old boy if you do them. Inversions are regularly cited as recipes for anti-aging, literally turning your body, and its clock, upside down. Although when you look at pictures of B. K. S. Iyengar, Krishnamacharya, and Desikachar, three of the foremost practitioners of "modern" yoga, you will see bodies that have indeed aged, all three remained vital and powerful into their old age (and Iyengar still is). Their internal organs remained youthful and healthy, even as the container aged.

Since doing yoga and strengthening the spleen meridian through energy medicine can both have a major impact on how we age, it only makes sense to combine the two practices.

The Liver Meridian: The Spleen's Special Partner

The liver meridian is on the control cycle with the spleen meridian, which means it helps to determine how much energy the spleen gets or releases. They are both yin meridians, which means they work constantly, without ceasing. The liver meridian is constantly flushing things out of the body, and the spleen meridian is constantly metabolizing.

These two meridians are often out of balance, and if they're not in harmony, they throw each other off. We've already talked about the importance of the spleen meridian, but the liver meridian is equally important. The liver is responsible for the smooth flow of chi in the body. The liver meridian is also associated with the smooth movement of emotions. When blood moves through the body in balanced flow, our emotions move with a smooth flow and don't get stuck.

The physical liver has more than seven hundred unique tasks that it's responsible for, and it is a primary player in the production and metabolization of hormones. (Hormones are produced by either amino acids or cholesterol, and cholesterol is produced in the liver.) It also processes toxins and poisons, stores energy in the form of glycogen, and aids the immune system. It governs ligaments and tendons, whose health is crucial to the physical body. The liver meridian makes sure the liver has enough energy to perform all its tasks.

Because the energy of the liver meridian is on the control cycle with the spleen meridian, it helps dictate the energy of the spleen, and when one is strong, the other tends to be deficient. Most often, the liver energy tends to be excessive, while spleen energy tends to be deficient—yet another reason why it's important for us to strengthen the spleen meridian.

Other Important Concepts: Meridian Strengthening, Sedating, and Control Points

We have built-in systems of the body that soothe, calm, and repattern the nervous system and many of the energy systems. There are specific acupoints, places where the meridian lines rise close to the surface of the body, that we can hold to help release trauma, help our immune system to function better, help calm the stress response, and help move pain out of the body. These are locations where there is a lower electrical resistance than in other areas. Donna Eden, David Feinstein, and Gary Craig, in their book *The Promise of Energy Psychology*, note that MRI studies have shown that "stimulating specific points on the skin not only *changed* brain activity; *it also deactivated areas of the brain that are involved with the experiences of fear and pain."*

These holds are simple to learn, and you can work with them in many different poses. As a general rule, sedating points are used to help relieve pain. Holding these points is like pulling the plug in a tub, allowing the water to run out, clearing the tub. The strengthening points are generally held when you want to infuse the meridian and the associated organ with more energy, like plugging the tub to fill it with fresh water. The control points are used to stop and solidify the process of either strengthening or sedating.

You'll notice the strengthening and sedating points for a meridian are actually located on two different meridians. For example, to strengthen the spleen meridian, you hold a point on the spleen meridian (spleen 2) and a point on the heart meridian (heart 8). The reason for this is related to the control and flow cycles of the meridians, how they relate to each other, and the fact that a different element controls each point on the meridian. (See week 5 for more on the five elements.) The specific points allow the meridian whose high tide precedes or follows the one you're working with to either give or take energy from that meridian. The points are chosen so that the different meridians can communicate more easily with one another.

Many of the practices we do in Energy Medicine Yoga help the energies in the body cross over from one side of the body to the other. Meridians, however, work in parallel lines, running up and down the body. Meridian strengthening and sedating points come in mirrored pairs. And you'll learn to hold these pairs *on the same side of the body,* one of the few non-crossed-over patterns.

I had a client who kept trying to sedate kidney to help with pain in his Achilles tendon (one of the uses of sedating a meridian is to alleviate pain). He complained it wasn't working. I checked how he was holding the points, and sure enough, he was crossing the points—holding one point on one side of the body and the other point on the opposite side—instead of holding both of the points on the same side of the body. As soon as he corrected this, he was able to ease his pain.

Practices of the Week: Working with the Triple Warmer, Spleen, and Kidney Meridians

The most important balancing thing you can do for your meridians on a regular basis is to balance the triple warmer and spleen meridians. For most people, this means calming triple warmer and strengthening the spleen meridian. I strengthen spleen every day, usually during my yoga practice, but I'll also do practices like the triple warmer–spleen hug while watching a movie, Skyping with a friend, or riding in a car (though not when I'm driving!). Balancing triple warmer and spleen is that important and that easy.

Working with the kidney and spleen meridians, the meridians that tend to weaken most with age, is also important for our overall vitality and wellbeing. So included in this week's practices is a forward-bend sequence that works with the kidney meridian, and one that strengthens the spleen meridian. Finally, you'll learn how a mudra you're probably already doing in your yoga practice is helping to boost your spleen meridian.

You can do all of these practices in your daily routine or rotate them. I'm going to show you the way I most often practice them, but feel free to take note of the meridian strengthening and sedating points and use them in any pose that seems best for your body or yoga practice.

THE TRIPLE WARMER–SPLEEN HUG

The triple warmer–spleen hug helps balance these two energies that otherwise can lead to feelings of overwhelm. Maintaining their balance can also help with weight issues, cravings, mood swings, and blood sugar imbalances.

Wrap your right arm around your body under your breast, so that your hand is resting on the left rib cage. Wrap your left hand around your body, with the left hand just above the right elbow. Hold just above the bend, on the outside of the arm. In this position, you are covering the spleen and triple warmer acupressure points; they will start to synch together, thereby listening to each other and being calmed by each other. If you tune into your hands while you're holding here, you can start to feel these two areas start to pulse together.

You can do this hug while standing in a line, sitting in front of the TV—anywhere really. Incorporating it into some yoga poses can help you ground more deeply, as well as keep the energy systems from being negatively impacted by the stress introduced by the yoga pose itself. One of my favorite uses of the triple warmer–spleen hug is in warrior I. We'll also use it in slow sit-ups.

SLOW SIT-UPS WITH THE TRIPLE WARMER–SPLEEN HUG

These sit-ups are different from your usual run-of-the-mill sit-ups, and I taught them to my military students with great results. Don't be discouraged if they seem impossible at the beginning. I've seen male cadets who can dead-lift two hundred pounds be unable to do even one. But the muscles learn this work very quickly, and you'll notice a rapid increase of strength if you practice these sit-ups regularly.

Lie on your back, with your knees bent, feet on the floor, hip width apart. The farther away your feet are from your body, the easier the sit-ups are, so adjust accordingly. If doing the sit-ups with bent knees is still too challenging, you can extend the legs all the way in front of you straight on the floor.

Wrap your arms around your torso in the triple warmer–spleen hug: right hand on the left rib cage, left hand holding right above the bend in the right elbow, on the outside of the arm.

Apply jalandhara bandha, tucking the chin in toward the throat. This will also help take the weight of the head off the neck and keep you from using your neck muscles in this posture. If you feel any strain in your neck, you can do these sit-ups with your head in your hands, being sure to soften the neck completely. You are using your stomach muscles and core strength, so be mindful.

Begin to slowly lift your body toward your bent knees. Do not use any momentum—that is the key to this posture. Go slow, slow, slow, using the deep core muscles. Press your belly down into the floor as you lift your body up toward your thighs. Come down with the same incredibly slow speed, making the muscles work on the down as much as the up. (See figure 15.) Apply mula bandha to help you tap into the deep core strength you need. Think about pushing down to lift up. If you get to a point where you cannot lift any farther without the feet popping up, stay at that point and keep pressing your stomach muscles toward the floor. Don't rock yourself up by pulling on your arms or cheating your feet off the floor. When you need to release, slowly lower down at the same speed. This point is your weakest-link spot, and if you muscle or momentum your way through it, it will stay your weakest link. As you breathe and strengthen slowly up to it, this link will get stronger. And you'll build that strength remarkably quickly.

If you incorporate these sit-ups into your practice consistently, you'll begin to notice a difference in a matter of days. These are super, super slow sit-ups. Generally you will work up to doing only five of them—they work that strongly.

Deep nose breathing allows the body to hold a stress-inducing position without provoking a stress response. The use of the triple warmer–spleen hug also keeps your body from experiencing stress in this pose. By adding the hug to the pose, you give the body one more tool to help it remain calm and to imprint itself with the energetic pathways of calm versus the pathways of stress.

THE HOOK UP: ALTERNATE VERSION, WORKING WITH THE BANDHAS

Working with the Hook Up, one of the energy medicine techniques that comprise the Wake Up sequence (see week 1), is another way to tap into the bandhas and triple warmer together. The Hook Up encourages the meridians that run around the core of the body to align and strengthen, which helps keep our core strong. It is indicated any time there is something structural or out of alignment with the spine, such as scoliosis, vertebral imbalances, back pain, or problems with posture. It also corresponds to our ability to support ourselves, to "stand up straight" and face our responsibilities.

You've learned the Hook Up with one finger in the belly button and one on the third eye. An alternate version is to have one finger in the belly button and one finger in the power point, the deep hollow at the center of the back of the head, where the head connects to the neck. Try both of these hand positions and see which induces a greater shift into calmness.

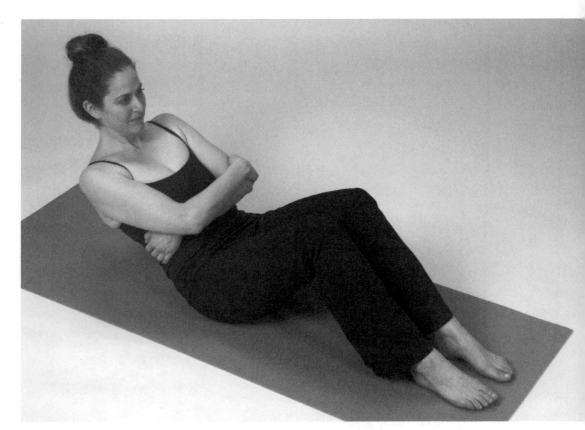

FIGURE 15   **Slow sit-up with triple warmer—spleen hug**

You can also experiment with applying deeper pressure in your belly button. If you reach in deeply and pull up, you are touching your diaphragm, the seat of uddiyana bandha and the middle burner of triple warmer. This can be a very tactile way to feel an upward lift in the body and to help you focus your attention at the navel center.

Donna Eden says she doesn't get out of bed in the morning without first hooking herself up. It is one of those quick energy medicine techniques that makes a huge difference in your overall feeling. The Hook Up helps to strengthen your aura, as well as to connect your yin and yang energies together. I encourage you to do a Hook Up several times during your Energy Medicine Yoga practice.

KIDNEY THREE-POINT POSE

This sequence works with the kidney meridian and comprises three seated floor poses and meridian-point holds:

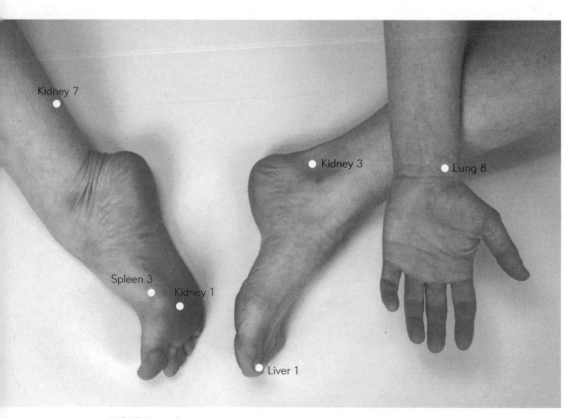

FIGURE 16   Points used in the Kidney Three-Point Pose

Kneeling spinal twist with kidney-sedating hold

Half ankle-to-knee pose (*ardha agnistambhasana*) with kidney-strengthening hold

Cobbler's pose (*baddha konasana*) with kidney-control-points hold

Figures 16 and 20 show all of the kidney sedating, strengthening, and control points.

Kneeling spinal twist with kidney-sedating hold. Kneel and sit back on your haunches. Allow the spine to be straight and lifted. Gently begin to twist to the right. Take your right hand and bring it to your right foot, pressing the thumb into the center of the ball of the foot. Wrap your fingers over the toes (the tops of which are touching the floor), and cover the point on the inside edge of the big-toe toenail. (See figure 17.)

Your thumb is on the first point of the kidney meridian (kidney 1), and your finger is holding the first point of the liver meridian (liver 1, see figure 20). Holding these points sedates the kidney meridian, flushing out stagnant energy and toxins. This hold is wonderful to do in twists—even a gentle twist like this one—as twists are also detoxifying.

Hold the points for two to three minutes. You'll start to feel a slight pulse, almost like a blood pulse, under these two points, and by about three minutes, they will synchronize. Release the points, slowly untwist, and repeat on the other side.

Kidney-sedating points exact locations (figures 16 and 20):

Kidney 1: Under the ball of the foot, almost in its exact center. Where the ball of the big toe and the ball of the other four toes meet, there is a slight indent.

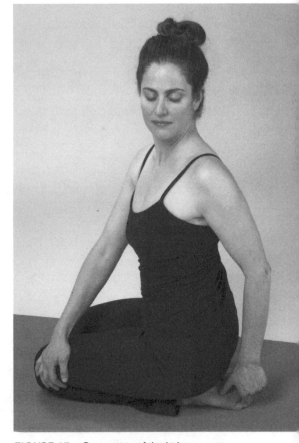

FIGURE 17   One option of the kidney-sedating hold, in kneeling spinal twist

Liver 1: On the base of the big-toe toenail, on the side closest to the pinky toe.

Tip: You can also hold the kidney-sedating points in half seated spinal twist (*ardha matsyendrasana*). If neither of these twists is possible for you, you can come into cobbler's pose and do all three holds here.

Half ankle-to-knee pose (ardha agnistambhasana) with kidney-strengthening hold. This pose is a very challenging hip opener, and you may want to start by sitting on the edge of a folded blanket or two, to raise the hips off the floor and help you keep your lower back straight.

Straighten your left leg and bend your right knee out to the side. Cross the ankle of the right foot above the left knee. (If your hips are more open, you can do this hold in the full pose: Stack your calves one on top of the other. Make sure your ankles are both flexed to protect both the knees and ankles.)

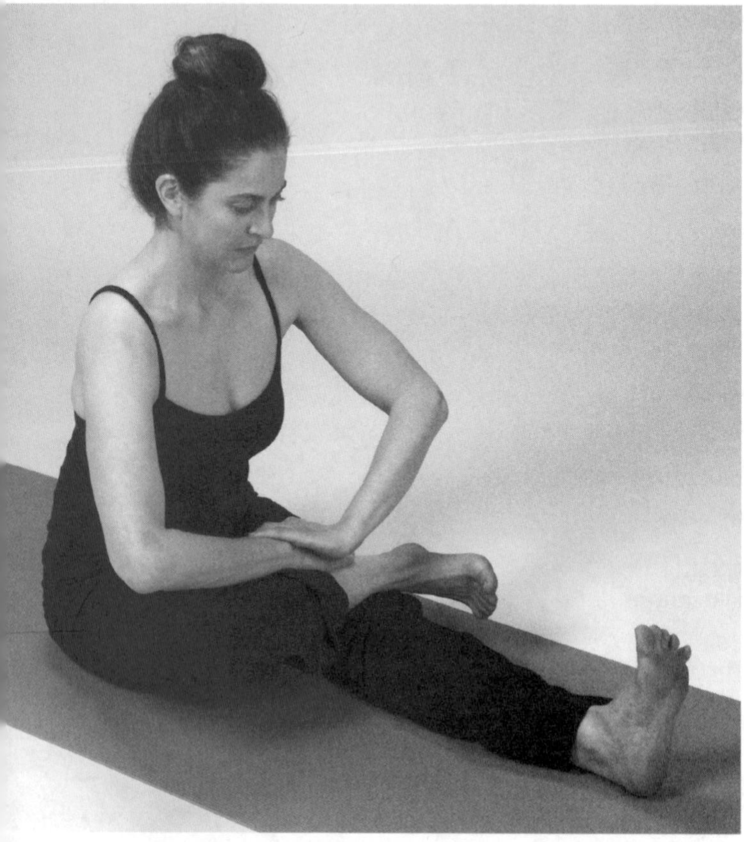

Now take your right hand and cover the point about one hand's breadth up the calf from the center of Achilles tendon (kidney 7) in line with the Achilles. Take your left hand and hold the thumb-side edge of the right wrist (lung 8). (See figure 18.) You don't have to worry about the exact location of the points; the wisdom of your body will find them. Hold them for about three minutes, and they will start to pulse together. I suggest using your whole hand to cover

FIGURE 18   Kidney strengthening hold in half ankle-to-knee pose

each point, to make sure you've got it. By holding these two points, you are strengthening the kidney meridian.

Hold for two to three minutes, then switch sides.

Kidney-strengthening points exact locations (figure 16):

Lung 8: Next to the ropey tendon on your inner wrist, on the side of your thumb. It is one finger span below the fold of your wrist.

Kidney 7: Behind the anklebone, find the center of the Achilles tendon, then go directly up the calf four finger widths.

Cobbler's pose (baddha konasana) with kidney-control-points hold. Sit on the floor with your legs extended in front of you; bend your knees out to the side and bring the soles of your feet together, coming into cobbler's pose. Put your thumbs directly in the center hollow of the Achilles tendon on both feet; you're holding both of the kidney 3 points. Stretch your first three fingers to the side of the ball of the foot and hold them on the downhill or heel-side edges; you're holding both spleen 3 points. These are the control points for kidney, and holding them balances the energy that you've just brought into the meridian with the previous two poses and holds in the sequence.

Begin to lean forward from the hips, keeping the back straight (figure 19). Hold for a minute and a half. (The control-points holds are half as long as the sedating or strengthening points.)

Kidney control points exact locations (figure 16):

Spleen 3: On the downward-sloping (toward the heel) outside edge of the ball of the foot.

Kidney 3: Directly behind the anklebone, in the center of the Achilles tendon.

Tip: If you want a more detailed description of locations of any of the points in these techniques, check out Acupressure.com.

When doing a three-point hold (the technique outlined above—holding a meridian's sedating, strengthening, and control points), we are essentially overhauling the meridian completely. We first clear it (sedate), then fill it (strengthen), then allow it to settle (control points). We don't always want to do this full technique on every meridian, and the reasons vary. For example, you never sedate the heart meridian, and you rarely strengthen triple warmer.

Our next technique is to strengthen the spleen meridian. Again, there are times when you might want to sedate the spleen meridian or do a three-point hold where you sedate spleen first, but the reasons for doing so are specific to a unique set of circumstances and individual energy needs of the moment. For our purposes here, we only want to strengthen the spleen.

HEAD-TO-KNEE POSE (*JANU SIRSASANA*) WITH SPLEEN STRENGTHENING

I like to do a spleen-strengthening hold in half-seated forward bend and full forward bend. Figure 20 provides a map of the spleen strengthening and control points used in this practice.

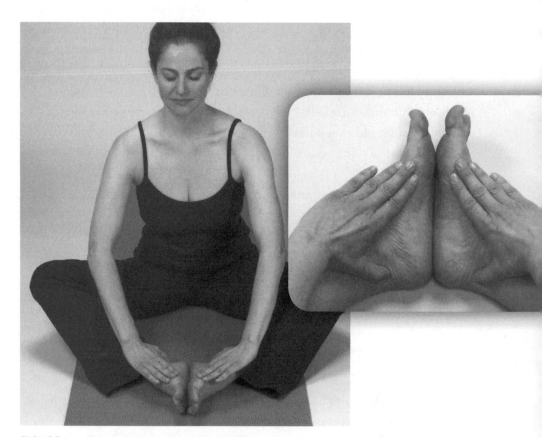

FIGURE 19   Kidney control points held in cobbler's pose

Begin seated. Lift your hips up by sitting on the edge of a folded blanket. Bend your right knee out to the side and place the sole of your right foot along the inside of the left leg. Inhale, lengthening out of your waist, lift your arms up overhead, and slowly exhale, folding over your legs, letting your arms drift with you, smoothing out the auric field. Inhale, curl the body back upright, and lengthen your arms up overhead. Exhale and fold again over your legs. Repeat the up-and-down movement a few times, to acclimate the body to the movement. When you feel ready, stay bent over your legs.

Now, in the bend, you're going to hold the first set of spleen-strengthening points.

If you're flexible enough to easily reach the foot of the extended left leg, you'll hold the points on the left side first. Take each finger of the left hand and thread it into the space between each toe, starting with the pinky finger between the pinky toe and fourth toe. Your thumb will be free to hold the second spleen meridian point on the ball of the foot (spleen 2). Then take the right hand and

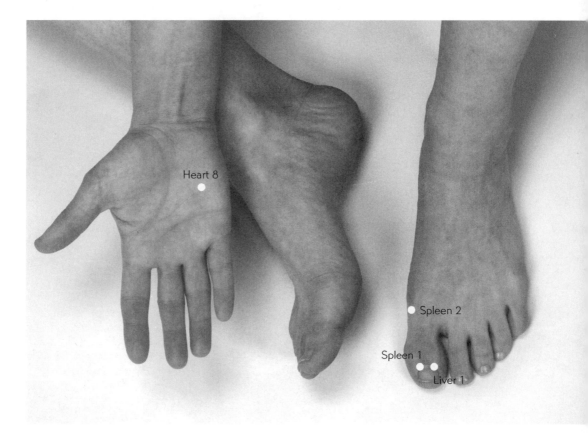

FIGURE 20   Spleen strengthening and control points

slide the right palm under the pinky side of the left hand. The eighth point on the heart meridian (heart 8) is located on the palm, between the fourth and fifth metacarpal bones. (When you make a fist, the point is where the tip of the little finger touches.) The fingers of your right hand will be resting on the heart 8 point of the left hand in this position. (See figure 21.)

If you can't bend forward far enough to easily reach your left foot, don't worry; you can work with the spleen-strengthening points on the bent right leg. Bring your right hand to the ball of the foot and hold the uphill slope, toward your toes (spleen 2). Now wrap the left hand over the pinky edge of the right hand, so that the left fingers curve around into the edge of your right palm to cover heart 8 on the right hand. (See figure 22.)

Whichever position you're in, stay there and continue to deepen your breath and your stretch as you hold the points. Pay attention to the points, and soon you will feel a slight pulsation under your fingers. After a minute or two, the pulsations should synchronize with each other. This is the spleen meridian

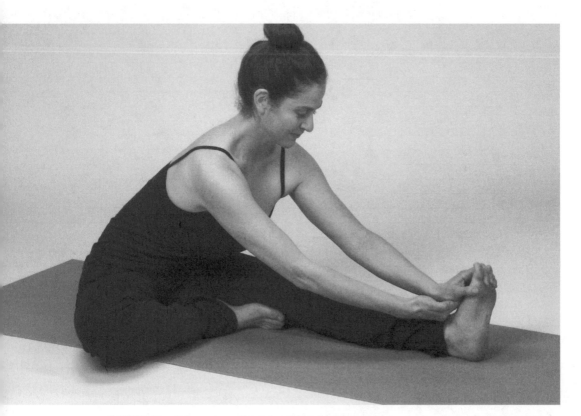

FIGURE 21   Spleen-strengthening points held in head-to-knee pose, advanced position

energy hooking up. You can continue to hold the pose and the points as long as you like, breathing evenly as you do. The longer you hold here, the deeper the stretch gets and the stronger the meridian charge becomes. I like to hold this pose three minutes or longer.

When you're ready to release, simply exhale, let go of the points, and sit back up. Straighten the bent leg and take a breath or two to adjust.

Repeat on the other side.

Spleen strengthening points exact locations (figure 20):

Heart 8: On the palm, between the fourth and fifth metacarpal
bones. When a fist is made, the point is where the tip of the little
finger touches.

Spleen 2: In front of the ball of the foot, toward the big toe, at the
outside edge where the skin of the sole and the top of the foot meet.

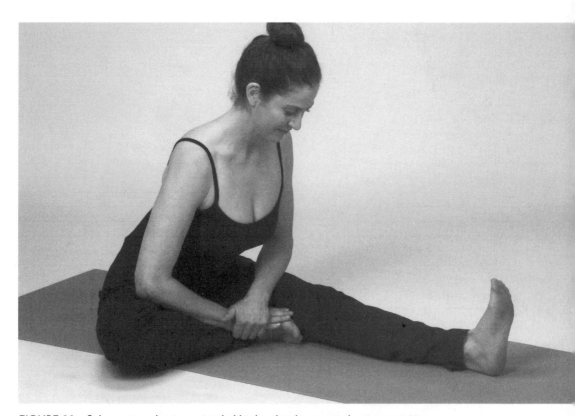

FIGURE 22   Spleen-strengthening points held in head-to-knee pose, beginner position

Cobbler's pose with spleen control points. When you've completed the spleen-strengthening hold on the second side, you are ready to hold the control points. This turns off the increase of energy to the meridian and stabilizes it.

Bring the soles of the feet together, knees out to the side. Sit up tall, lifting the torso out of the hips, and lean forward from the low belly (not the upper body). While sitting in cobbler's pose, place the first two fingers of each hand on the bottom corners of each big-toe toenail. The first point on the spleen meridian (spleen 1) is located on the bottom outer edge of the toenail (the edge closest to the arch of the foot). The first point of the liver meridian (liver 1) is located on the bottom inner edge of the toenail (the edge closest to the pinky-toe side of the foot).

Lean forward, and breathe. You can hold this pose for one to two minutes, and you will also begin to feel the points pulsing together, hooking up.

When you feel complete, inhale, and sit up.

Tip: If you are more flexible, you can hold the control points in full forward bend (*pashimottanasana*), with both legs straight out in front of you (figure 23).

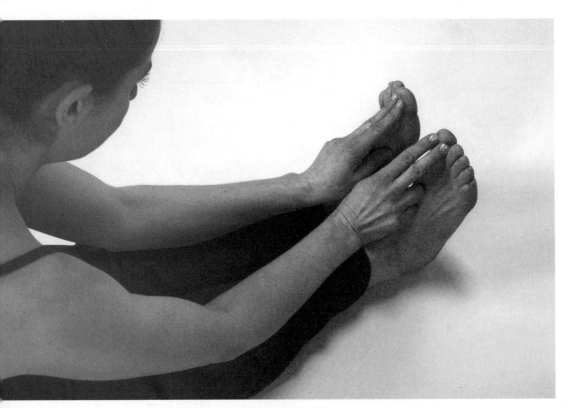

FIGURE 23   Spleen control points held in full forward bend

YOGIC TOE LOCK

If you have practiced yoga for a while, you have used the very powerful spleen-strengthening points—spleen 1 and liver 1—unwittingly in the yogic toe lock. In this lock, you hold the big toe with the first two fingers and thumb. As explained earlier, the liver and spleen meridians have a symbiotic relationship, and holding these two points boosts the spleen while calming the liver. Liver 1, the first point on the liver meridian, located at the base of the big toenail, is known as "the etheric point of the whole body." Accessing this point helps you open to the etheric field, the part of the aura that holds the essence of your spirit, as well as the blueprint for your body. It is the innermost layer of your aura.

These two points, held and pressed in concert with each other, form a powerful dance of healing and building resiliency and adaptability, as well as help to balance the hormones. When I learned the importance of holding these points together in energy medicine, I was again impressed with the wisdom of the ancient yogis and wanted to reintroduce the energetic importance of this mudra to my yoga students.

The yogic toe lock is used in many poses: leg extensions while standing, forward bends with the legs together or apart, and seated forward bends. In virtually any pose where you might reach and hold onto your foot, use this hold.

COBBLER'S POSE (BADDHA KONASANA) WITH GAIT CLEARING

After doing kidney- and spleen-meridian work, I like to clear the energy gaits in the toes again. Clearing the toe gaits helps to clear the liver, since the liver meridian runs down between the big toe and the second toe and ends at the base of the big-toe toenail.

Return to cobbler's pose. Using your fingers and thumbs, firmly massage along the metatarsal bones that separate each toe. Be sure to pinch off in the gully between the toes, opening up the energy channels and releasing constricted energy. You can also massage and pinch the tip of each toe.

Then squeeze both sides of the feet and give a firm massage to the instep bone on the upward-facing interiors of both feet. The bones that start from the top of the big toe, rise up at the arch, and end at the heel bone mimic the spine, and in reflexology, these bones are massaged to help release spinal tension.

If you want to stay in cobbler's pose a bit longer, you can also clear the hand gaits and then vigorously shake excess energy off the hands before coming out of the pose.

The Five Elements and the Power of Sound

This week we discuss the transformative power of sound in Energy Medicine Yoga and introduce a practice that links you to the seasons and the physical world through the five elements of TCM. This system is how our individual energy expresses itself in physical form.

Chanting and Speaking: The Power of Sound

When I taught yoga at a military university, chanting Sanskrit mantras was not the most obvious thing to do. For yoga teachers who teach in churches, community centers, or gyms, it may be a challenge to introduce the incredibly potent use of sound vibration to the class without offending some of the students' sensibilities or crossing over the rules or boundaries of the teaching venue. But do not let this discourage you from accessing this powerful tool for transformation. In your own personal practice, if you do not use some form of sound or vibration, please consider adding it.

Pandit Rajmani Tigunait, the spiritual head of the Himalayan Institute, writes about the use of sound in *The Power of Mantra and the Mystery of Initiation:* "Personality, speech, emotions, and the sense of attraction or repulsion are a few of the ways in which the life-force radiates from us. We also radiate different degrees and shades of light, sound, electricity, magnetism, and gravitational energy. Every cell of the body has its own vibratory pattern and, based on this pattern, sound waves emerge from each cell. But all the cells in an organism must function in a coordinated manner, they must all vibrate within a specific spectrum."

Chanting helps to entrain the cells—to create a cohesive pattern in the physical body by harmonizing the cell bodies.

The science of cymatics is the study of vibration made visible. You can go online and look at numerous experiments that illuminate the power of sound. In one, a high-fidelity speaker is placed underneath a metal tray on which sand is scattered. The speaker then produces a sustained tone. After a few moments, the sand miraculously shifts into a geometric pattern. As the tones rise in pitch, the patterns of the sand continue to switch, in instant, jumplike phases, becoming more and more sophisticated and complex. It is incredible to watch the beautiful patterns that emerge simply with the application of sound.

The following is excerpted from pioneering sound healer Eileen McKusick's book *Tuning the Human Biofield: Healing with Vibrational Sound Therapy* (Healing Arts Press, 2014):

> The human body is wired to be exquisitely sensitive to sound. The faculty of hearing is one of the first senses to develop in utero, and the last to depart before death. In addition to perceiving sound through our ears, the journal *Nature* recently published a paper (November 26, 2009 issue) detailing a NIH study that shows that we also "hear" the pressure waves of sound through our skin. Water, of which our bodies are largely composed, conducts sound at a rate approximately four times faster than air.
>
> Our bones also conduct sound, as evidenced by newer hearing aids that conduct sound through the skull directly to the cochlea.
>
> It has been discovered that in addition to the well-known *lock and key* structure of receptors on cell membranes that receive and respond to physical molecules, there are also *antenna-like structures* that respond to vibrational frequencies. Bruce Lipton writes in *The Biology of Belief* (2005):
>
> "Receptor antennas can also read vibrational energy fields such as light, sound, and radio frequencies. The antennas on these energy receptors vibrate like tuning forks. If an energy vibration in the environment resonates with a receptor's antenna, it will alter the protein's charge, causing the receptor to change shape. Because these receptors can read energy fields, the notion that only physical molecules can impact cell physiology is outmoded. Biological behavior can be controlled by invisible forces as well as it can be controlled by physical molecules like penicillin, a fact that provides the scientific underpinning for pharmaceutical-free energy medicine."

Conscious and intentional use of the human voice in chanting, singing, and toning has been used for millennia, often within a religious or devotional context. Numerous studies have been done to determine what exactly happens when we chant or sing or tone, whether alone or in groups. Neurological imaging has shown changes in blood flow to the brain, in addition to other biological markers of increased well-being, when experienced meditators are engaged in chanting meditation (Lazar, 2000). One study noted a positive emotional effect and immune competence as determined by the presence of secretory immunoglobulin A in saliva swabs after a choir rehearsal, and even more marked increase after a performance (Kreutz et al., 2006).

The process of toning, which has gained some popularity in recent years, is a sort of informal chanting where the individual simply intones extended vowel sounds that are supposed to help release energy blockages from the body. Chanting is said to have a similar result of facilitating the flow of energy through the body.

Another powerful and scientific reason to use sound in your Energy Medicine Yoga practice is the effect it has on the vagus nerve. This nerve is one of the longest nerves in the body, starting at the base of the cranium and taking a wandering path through the body before ending in the abdomen. It controls a variety of functions, including the heart rate and breathing. It also relays information from the digestive system to the brain. The digestive system is frequently referred to as "the second brain," because of the hundreds of millions of neurons embedded in the gut wall. The microbes in the gut wall manufacture 95 percent of our body's serotonin, a neurotransmitter responsible for feelings of happiness and wellbeing. Many stress-related chemicals are also produced in the gut, and these chemicals can alter the serotonin levels, disrupting the production of positive-mood-supporting chemicals. The vagus nerve is part of the complex dance between our gut brain and head brain. Finally, the vagus nerve is involved in physical functions in the throat, larynx, and ears.

Chanting and toning have been proven to stimulate the vagus nerve and to facilitate feelings of wellbeing. If you have never chanted or toned before, a good way to start is to use the sound *ah* and hold it as long as you can. To continue, you can tone the sound *ooh,* then *mmmm.* In my classes, I challenge my students to see who can hold the note the longest. This competition allows them to tone without feeling strange or awkward. After going through the vowel sounds in the alphabet, they are all fairly humming with the resonance and quite pleased with themselves. Chanting also helps to deepen your breath and concentrate your focus.

The sound of *OM* or *AUM* is considered the primordial sound of the universe, from which everything emerged. It is the "word" that God spoke to cause everything to come into being. It is also considered to be the waking, dreaming, and dreamless states of consciousness, or the generating energy (A), organizing energy (U), and destroying energy (M) of the universe.

It is a good practice to begin and end every Energy Medicine Yoga session with three OMs. You can practice chanting OM while coming into or out of deep forward bends or while standing in a balance pose. This fulfills many purposes: it adds the power of vibration to the practice, brings in an open-mouthed exhale, and creates an intense internal focus.

Sanskrit, the language of yoga, is a resonant language that affects the body, harmonizing and opening up energies. "Sanskrit is also the language of mantra, word formulas that were discovered by the ancient sages of India as being a particular combination of sound vibrations that, when chanted or meditated upon, had a specific result on the mind, psyche, or even the natural realm," notes Aja, president of the Atma Institute, in his online essay "Sanskrit: The Language of the Gods." So even if you don't know what the Sanskrit words mean, they have a transformative effect on the body. Each cell membrane in our bodies is alive with antenna-like structures that respond to vibration. By using this language that is attuned to opening up energy flows in the body, you are not only getting steeped in the yoga tradition through its language, but also tuning your energy to a higher vibration.

Energy System of the Week: The Five Elements

Our lives run in cycles. We have our daily cycle of wake, work, recreate, eat, sleep. We have the weekly cycle of work, school, commitments, weekends. We have the annual cycle of the seasons and holidays. If you're a woman, you have a monthly menstrual cycle. Our breath has a cycle—one that favors one nostril over the other for ninety minutes at a stretch. Each of these cycles has a rhythm and a time element to it, as well as a specific purpose: to rejuvenate (the sleep, hormonal, or menstrual cycles), to educate (the school-year cycle), to energize and calm (the breath cycle).

The cycle of the seasons is also purposeful for us. It is a constant reminder of both the renewal of life and the end of life. The seasons teach us about growth, abundance, decay, and death in a continual, ever-changing pattern. The cycle starts with the cold, dark, and wet of winter, where everything is still and inward focused. It is both a time of cessation and a time of gestation. This is followed by spring, a cycle of messy, wet, muddy brown earth, followed by bursts of greenery and new life, the outer manifestation of seeds' winter growth. Summer is the time of ripening and burning, hot and fiery. This is followed by autumn, the season of both harvest and decline.

In energy medicine as taught by Donna Eden, the five elements of TCM—water, wood, fire, earth, and metal—play a large and important role. Each person has a primary element, which, like the *doshas* in Ayurveda, is aligned with a particular season and forms a blueprint that overlays a person's behavior, choices, and lifestyle, as well as his or her psychology. This primary element is the lens through which you operate in the world, as well as the lens through which you get ill and heal from illness. For example, if your primary element is water, the themes that run through your life are new beginnings, new ideas, philosophy, and symbolism. Water people can be childlike, curious, and endearing, but also selfish and tactless. Their downfalls are fearfulness, suspicion, and negativity. Water governs the bones, fluids (except the blood), and teeth. So water people may find the tendency to illness or injury in those areas of their body.

Water, wood, earth, and metal each have two meridians that govern them, a yin and a yang meridian; fire, the fifth element, has four. Each element also has emotions that correlate with it. The yin-meridian emotion is a more inward-turning expression of the emotion, while the yang is a more outward-looking expression of the same emotion. Each of the five elements is also connected with one of the seasons.

In Energy Medicine Yoga, we follow the Eden Energy Medicine five-element season cycle based on TCM:

Winter/water. The challenging emotions are fear and shame. The balancing emotions are courage, trust, and gentleness with self.

Spring/wood. The challenging emotions are rage against yourself, general anger, and judgment. The balancing emotions are tolerance, kindness, certainty, and assertiveness.

Summer/fire. The challenging emotions are heartache, anxiety, and panic. The balancing emotions are discernment, peace, inspiration, and joy.

Solstice and equinox/earth. The challenging emotions are over-compassion and excessive worry. The balancing emotions are compassion for self and sympathy.

Autumn/metal. The challenging emotions are grief, the desire to control, and holding on. The balancing emotions are letting go, inspiration, and faith.

Originally the Chinese five elements were four elements arranged around a cross. Earth was in the center, and each season would come back to the center and reground itself before moving to the next season and element. You can see the elegance of this, as the solstices and equinoxes mark the change of the four seasons. And both the cross and the number four are balanced. At some point in the development of TCM, earth was moved to the outside of the circle, and the seasonal flow that we see today was put into place.

We are all prone to imbalance in our lives. Every single action you do takes the body out of homeostasis, and the goal of any health practice, including yoga and energy medicine, is to bring it back. Balance is a constant dance, an art form really, rather than any specific or static location. During a yoga practice, you see that the most clearly with the power of the balancing poses. You are constantly making micro-adjustments to your body, the bandhas, and the breath, in order to maintain balance.

Just as being out of balance physically can make us fall over when we're practicing tree pose (*vrksasana*), being out of balance mentally or emotionally can make us fall out of the flow of our daily lives. If our diet is too stressful on the digestive system, or our work lives require too much energy, or our emotional lives are draining instead of nourishing, we can feel overwhelmed and fall out of our place of balance and contentment. If these imbalances get large enough, they can lead to injury and disease, forcing us to abandon our activities and reevaluate our routines.

Stress is such a big part of our lives and is now recognized to be the leading cause of most disease. Stress can be caused by any number of factors, but one of the biggest culprits is our inability to process emotions when they occur. Most of us have had experiences where we feel overwhelmed by our emotions, whether they are fear, anger, anxiety, or the inability to let go of things. Even the feeling of compassion can overwhelm us, especially when we think about the state of the world and the suffering of so many people. Undigested emotions are what set up our problems, as they throw off our biologic systems. Working with the five-elements flow is a way to continually release and calm our emotional body.

The five elements comprise a complex and powerful energy system that, once understood, helps to illuminate the rest of the energy systems. The five elements are about movement and change. Everything changes because energy wants to move, so our goal is to stay in dynamic movement with the shifting tides. The five elements are woven through all the energy systems. They are like a pattern that overlays each of our unique energy systems, with a beat or an accent on our specific element. Our personalities and our tendencies toward certain imbalances are intimately connected with one or two of the five elements. Our connection to the natural world and the seasons of the year is also reflected in these elements. The challenge is that we generally only see the five-elements energy system when it is out of balance. When it is in balance, we are resilient.

It can be helpful, and fun, to know what your primary and secondary element are. There are many simple five-elements quizzes you can find online to help determine this. Once you know, you may find it helpful to practice your specific elemental movement on a more regular basis if the issues connected with that element resonate with you.

The five-elements system offers a huge body of wisdom, more than we can go into here, and can seem enormous with all its variables and possible combinations. But once learned and understood, it provides a powerful tool for diagnosing and treating specific disorders, as well as for keeping the whole body-mind complex balanced and healthy in relation to the environment and the cyclical nature of life.

Practice of the Week: The Five-Elements Salutation

Donna Eden has written extensively about the five elements, and created unique movement and breath exercises for each one. I've taken those exercises and, with her permission, woven them into one continuous flow—a five-element emotional-release *vinyasa,* or series of flowing postures. The five elements are the meridians in relationship, and doing this flow helps to balance the emotions as well as the energetic systems. It also helps to balance out the extremities of the seasons. Donna sees energy, and when I showed her the five-element salutation, she remarked on the beautiful transformation of energy around my body. She saw how the energy changed from start to finish.

Any one of the individual elemental exercises can be taken out of this flow and practiced by itself, as Donna teaches, if you feel you need more of its specific benefits. For example, in summer, which is the season of fire, many people feel they're burning out of control, full of anxiety for everything they need to do and fix and participate in. This is fire in its unhealthy state. This is wildfire burning out of control. The exercise called Bringing Down the Flame helps to re-educate the fire and seat it in the solar plexus, where you want the fire to be. This is the fire in the belly. This is the place of power and inspiration, burning up your toxins, feeding your willpower so you can accomplish and achieve what you need to, and inspiring you to burn brightly and be a light in the world. In summer, or when you're feeling anxious, perhaps you will add only the fire exercise to your practice.

Otherwise, to keep you in a healthy balance, I recommend you do the entire five-element salutation daily. Cycling through the seasons of the year and the emotions every day will keep you in balance.

Each element has a corresponding sound, and toning that sound will help you release the emotions connected with the element. These sounds were discovered by ancient practitioners of TCM. Each organ and meridian has a sound, and the element sounds are derived from those.

I'm going to first describe the reasons and meaning behind each movement, then give you the instructions for doing them all together.

THE SEASONS, THEIR ELEMENTS, AND THEIR EMOTIONS

Winter. The element is water, and the challenging emotion is fear. The yin meridian is kidney, and the yang meridian is bladder. Winter is the start of the seasonal cycle, and as such, it is like a young child, uncertain, unsure, feeling isolated and alone. The fear is the primal fear of the dark. The movement for this season is called Blowing Out the Candle, and by doing this movement, you move from fear to courage and trust—trust that even in the darkness of this deep-growth season, you are safe and protected.

Spring. Spring's element is wood, and the challenging emotion is anger. The yin meridian is liver, and the yang meridian is gallbladder. The spring movement is called Expelling the Venom, and once the venom is expelled there is no anger or righteousness. In its negative aspect, anger is that feeling that nothing is right, nothing is going well. You're like a car stuck in the mud of the spring rains, unable to move forward. But releasing and transforming this anger brings about the power of the wood element of spring—the power of a plant shoot that breaks through the concrete in the sidewalk. People who see the world from the point of view of the wood element are powerful manifestors. They understand that there are things in the world that are theirs, and they take them. They don't take in a greedy way; there is no grasping or hoarding. It is just the confident understanding of what is theirs. They ask for and get the raise they deserve because they deserve it. Theirs is the power of the tree that bends in the storm but stays rooted and strong in the place that belongs solely to that tree. They take their rightful place in the world.

Summer. The element for summer is fire. The yin meridians are heart and circulation-sex. The yang meridians are triple warmer and small intestine. In balance, summer is excitement and inspiration. Out of balance, it is anxiety. In the summer movement, called Bringing Down the Flame, we re-educate the out-of-control fire by drawing the energy from around and outside of us, into the spinal column, or Sushumna, where the chakras can temper the wildness of the season. Lastly, we seat the fire in the naval center where it can work for us instead of against us.

Solstice and equinox. The element is earth, and the challenging emotion is over-compassion. The yin meridian is spleen, and the yang meridian is stomach. The movement for these pivot points between seasons is called Cradling the Baby. Sometimes we feel so deeply the pain of everyone around us, even the pain of the whole world, that we try to do everything we can to help everyone we know, but the end result is that often we burn ourselves out in the process. Many people who do body work or healing arts or who are parents or caretakers find themselves in this position. They give until they give out. The balance comes when we turn that over-compassion for others into deep compassion for ourselves. The first rule of first aid is to make sure *you're* okay. You can't help anyone else unless you are balanced and stable and your cup is full.

Autumn. The element is metal, and the challenging emotion is grief. The yin meridian is lung, and the yang meridian is large intestine. The autumn path is the path of letting go and having the wisdom to know what is necessary to hold onto and what is necessary to release. To transform grief into its more powerful and balanced component, letting go, we need to surrender our belief that we are in control and that we know everything. Whatever your belief system is, it is a huge relief to surrender to the truth that sometimes you simply do not know the best path and that you simply cannot be responsible for everything. The autumn movement is called Human Touching Divine.

THE PRACTICES (IN SEQUENCE)

Blowing Out the Candle (winter). Start in a squat, with your arms wrapped around your knees. You can have your heels propped on a blanket to help support you. If you don't feel comfortable yet in this full, deep squat, you can start in a chair, with your torso folded forward and arms wrapped around your knees.

Bow your head. Inhale, lift the head up, and exhale through pursed lips, as if you're blowing out a candle in front of you (figure 24). Make the sound *whhhoooo* as you exhale. Curl your head down again, take a deep inhale, lift your head up, and blow out the candle again with a *whhhoooo* sound. Do this once more.

Expelling the Venom (spring). From the squat or seated position at the end of Blowing Out the Candle, release your arms from around your legs and come up into chair pose. If you're doing this pose on its own, simply come into chair pose. Drop your hands in front of you and make each hand into a fist. Grab into those fists all your fear and all your anger. Circle your arms first around behind you and then up over your head. With a strong *shhhh* sound, throw your fists down toward the ground, opening them up and emptying them onto the earth (figure 25). Do this again. Grab the junk, the fear, the anger, the rage—whatever is holding you back—circle it around and up, and then throw it down to the ground with a strong *shhhh*. Do this one last time, but this time, move slowly, with intention, as you grab your emotions and throw them down, expelling them with a strong *shhhh*.

Bringing Down the Flame (summer). Stand straight up in tadasana, with your hands on the front of your thighs. Take a deep inhale and exhale with the sound *haaa*. Feel a grounding energy building in your hands and going down your legs into the earth.

Inhale, and circle your hands overhead, bringing them together so that all the fingers and the thumbs are touching. Exhale with

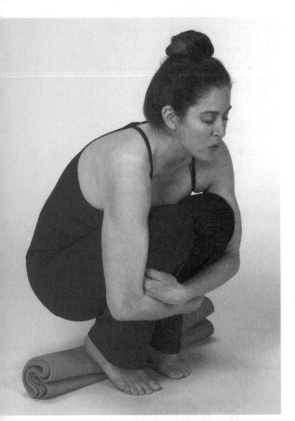

FIGURE 24   **The Five Elements Salutation: Blowing Out the Candle**

the *haaa* sound and bring the thumbs down to the top of the head, the center of the crown chakra (figure 26). You are bringing the wild, out-of-control fire element into the wisdom and strength of your crown chakra, your connection to the divine. Think about pouring the fire down into the spinal column, the core of the nervous system, as well as the energetic core of the body. You are realigning this fire with the intelligence of the chakras, which reach into this central channel.

Release your hands from the crown of the head and circle them around again on an inhale. Exhale with the sound *haaa* and bring the fingers and thumbs together, this time with the thumbs touching the middle of the forehead. With this movement, you are re-educating the fire by aligning it to the third eye, which is your inner spiritual connection, your intuition.

Again, release the hands and circle them around, exhaling with the *haaa* and bringing the thumbs to the heart center. Here you are re-educating the fire by aligning it with love, both giving and receiving.

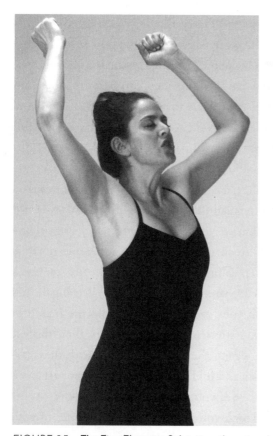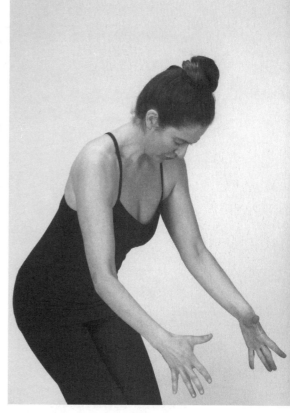

FIGURE 25   **The Five Elements Salutation: throwing down your anger in Expelling the Venom**

Inhale, circle the arms again, and bring the thumbs to the navel. This is where the fire wants to be seated, in the navel center. Exhale with the *haaa* sound, keeping your thumbs there, and tent your fingers so the pinky edges are resting on the pubic bone. Inhale, exhale with the *haaa* sound, and flatten the hands onto the low belly, keeping the index fingers and thumbs connected. This position is empowering the fire to burn strong over the first three chakras, where we generally have the densest layers of energy.

Inhale, and smooth your hands down the inside of your legs, then down and off the insides of the feet, shaking them off in front of you. Then exhale with the *haaa* sound, drawing the hands up the insides of the legs. From the groin, trace out at the hips, move up the outside of the body to the armpits, and come back down the sides, buzzing the spleen-meridian points.

Note: You may have noticed that we skip the throat chakra in Bringing Down the Flame. Donna sees the throat chakra as a series of chambers corresponding to each chakra, and it functions much like the sorting hat in the Harry Potter books, deciding what incoming energetic information should go to which chakra. We skip this chakra here because we don't want fire energy to become more complicated or have to go into a "sorting hat," but rather, we want to guide it onto a more calming and easeful path.

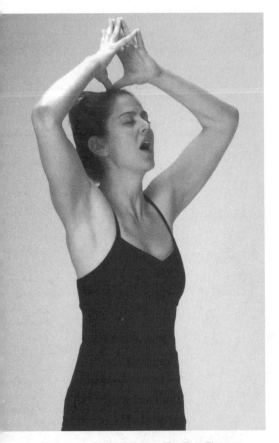

FIGURE 26   **The Five Elements Salutation: Bringing Down the Flame**

Cradling the Baby (solstice and equinox). Stand in tadasana and slide your hands around your midsection so you're giving yourself a hug (figure 27). Rock yourself side to side while inhaling and exhaling with the ujjayi breath (see week 3). Hug yourself for a bit, and then inhale and reach your arms overhead. Hold the breath in as you stretch the right arm up, then the left, right again, then the left. Exhale with the ujjayi breath and fold forward, reaching your arms out in front of you, into a full forward bend.

Reach your hands under the arches of your feet, either from the front or sides of your feet, and pull up your torso, away from your feet, straightening your arms and lifting your butt into the air. Exhale, and release your hands from beneath the feet. Inhale, and stand back up, tracing up the insides of your legs, out at the hips, up into your armpits, and down to the spleen points at the side of your ribs. Buzz the spleen points. Continue smoothing your hands under and around your breasts and then move them up until both hands are over your heart center, one on top of the other. Take another ujjayi breath.

Human Touching Divine (autumn). From tadasana with hands at the heart center, inhale, then exhale with a *sssss* sound as you release your hands to your thighs. Inhale and take a slight backbend, opening up your hands at the level of your hips (figure 28). Visualize yourself taking in the whole world around you, imagining all the people you love, all the people in your tribe, and then taking in the whole universe.

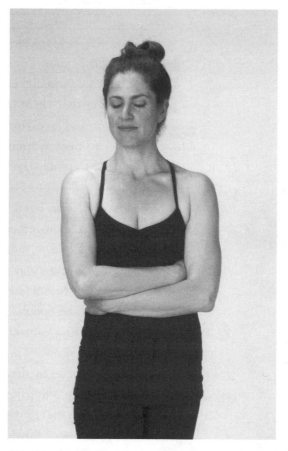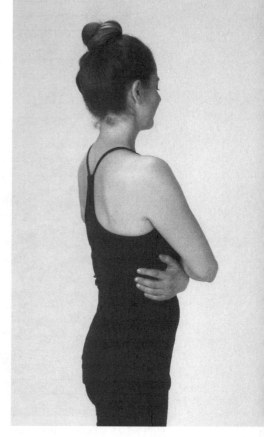

FIGURE 27   **The Five Elements Salutation: Cradling the Baby**

Exhale with a *ssss* sound and bring your hands forward, rounding your arms as though you were hugging a large beach ball in front of you. Your palms face toward your body, and your fingers are almost, but not quite, touching. Within the circle of your arms, imagine everyone in your world whom you love, and all the world and its grief and pain.

Inhale again and take a slightly higher backbend, your arms opening up around the level of your waist. This backbend is slightly higher in the spine. Feel as if you are letting everything go. It isn't your responsibility to heal all the trials and tribulations of the world.

Exhale with the *ssss* sound and bring your fingertips close, but not touching. Your arms are in front of your chest here. Feel as if you are Adam on the Sistine Chapel ceiling and God is reaching down to you. Feel that inexorable joy that comes when the divine spirit is indeed reaching out for you.

Inhale again, this time taking a full backbend, with your arms either shoulder height or above your head. Release everything to a higher power, trusting that there is a bigger plan and a divine intelligence at play. Surrender your need to understand or control.

Exhale with the *ssss* sound, bringing your hands together in front of and above your forehead, only this time allow the fingers to touch. Smooth your hands over the opposite arms, as if gathering yourself into a hug, and bring your hands to your chest, so they are crossed, resting one palm on each side of the upper chest over your lungs. Inhale and exhale the *ssss* sound.

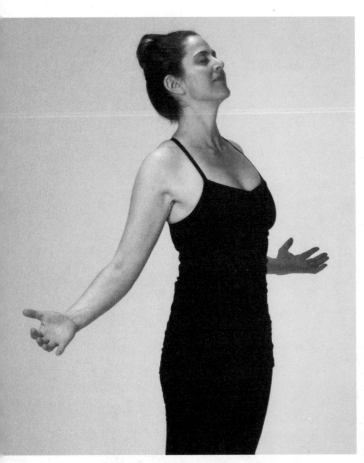

FIGURE 28   **The Five Elements Salutation: Human Touching Divine**

Take several deep breaths, exhaling with the *ssss* sound; alternately hold dear what you love and let go and surrender in faith.

Note: When I started experimenting with the Five-Elements Salutation, I loved doing it, and I could really feel how the sound helped me release emotion with each pose as I cycled through. But it was not until I went through a period of deep and unexpected grief that this vinyasa, especially the autumn practice, revealed its power to me. I did the autumn practice several times a day, and I found myself often just sitting or standing with my hands over my lungs, making the *ssss* sound. Sometimes for hours, I would just cry in a *ssss*. I didn't know why this sound was helping (this was before I knew where the sounds derived from), but the sound itself seemed to dissipate my grief. Also, crying, the release of tears, is important. Tears are the fluid of the liver. When under stress, we cry, and this releases excess hormones from our body in the tears themselves, relieving pressure on the liver. Crying is a biological tool and not to be seen as weakness or over-emotionality. Grief comes in waves and at unexpected times. I used the *ssss* over and over again to help move the grief out of my body. You can use the sounds of the elements to release emotions anytime and in any pose. They are powerful and easy tools to work with.

After you do the entire Five-Elements Salutation a couple of times, you can begin to do it more quickly. You don't need to stop at every motion and think through the feeling process. You can simply move the body, make the sounds, and let the power of this flow reveal itself to you.

Pranayama: Alternate Nostril Breath (*Nadi Shodanam*)

This breath is calming and balancing. By switching nostrils consciously, you help to balance the hemispheres of the brain. This technique is good to use if you're feeling overwhelmed, stressed, tired, or anxious, as it brings you back into a balanced state.

Since this is the week we're working on balancing our emotional bodies, it makes sense to start to use this breath here. If you take a few minutes to practice this breath prior to doing the Five-Element Salutation, you will increase even more your ability to process and smooth out the emotional ripples that are throwing you off your game. You can do this breath practice before or after your physical practice.

Bring your right hand to your nose with the first two fingers bent into the palm, into *vishnu mudra.* The ring finger and thumb will be on either side of the nose.

Inhale through both nostrils. Close the right nostril with the thumb, making sure you're pressing right up against the bone at the top of the nostril, and exhale through the left.

Inhale through the left nostril, and close off the left nostril with the ring finger, again touching the bone. Exhale through the right nostril.

Continue this pattern. Inhale, exhale, switch. Inhale, exhale, switch. If your hand gets tired, you can hold up the right elbow with the left hand, or place the first two fingers of the right hand on the third eye to help hold up the arm.

Continue this breath for several minutes.

When you feel complete, finish with an exhale from the left nostril. Allow the right hand to come back to your lap and your breathing to return to normal.

Sit quietly for a few minutes before moving.

MENTAL ALTERNATE NOSTRIL BREATH (*PRANA SHUDDHI*)

This breath is the same as above, but instead of using your fingers to close the nostrils, you simply imagine the breath ascending through one nostril and descending out the other.

Again, you'll start with the left nostril. See the breath, one to two inches from the end of the nose, rising up the left nostril into the midbrain. Then exhale and see the breath descending out the right nostril. Putting a color onto the breath can help the visualization. Notice how, as you continue, you can actually feel the breath move in one side and then out the other.

When you feel complete, exhale through the left nostril and relax, letting your breathing return to normal.

These two breaths, while helping balance the hemispheres of the brain, also balance the nadis of Ida and Pingala, bringing the energy into Sushumna, or spinal column (see week 2). Alternate nostril breath is used to balance these nadis, bringing the prana into the central column. Again, the balance of left and right, and drawing into the centerline, is emphasized here.

Empowered Warrior Series and the Electrics

This week you'll learn a different kind of warrior series and another way of working with visualization. You'll also learn how to get into the electrical system of the body. Hooking in to this energy system, which is the most physically tangible of all the energy systems, after working with the energy of the warrior, can help bring your intentions into a more visceral place, bringing them one step closer to reality.

Empowerment the Apache Way

By now you've done a bit of visualization and you're hopefully getting a deeper understanding of its power. Maybe you visualized smoothing your meridians this morning and immediately felt your energy moving. Maybe you visualized one of the radiant circuit flows and felt a surge of joy. Now I want to add one more component to your visualization practice.

I took a long break from teaching yoga in the middle of my career—a full seven years off. Soon after I stopped teaching, I met Donna Eden and began studying her energy medicine work on my own, but it would be another bunch of years before I enrolled in her formal program. During that interim time, I found myself immersed in the world of Tom Brown, Jr., and his primitive skills. I went to his tracker school, first in California and later in New Jersey, where I learned to make a fire using friction, build a warm shelter with leaves and sticks, track animals and learn their daily habits, build a bow by hand, flint knap stones, tan animal hides, and most profoundly, meditate like an Apache warrior. Tom's guiding force was the time he spent with Grandfather, an Apache Indian whom Tom had met as a young boy. Tom spent a dozen years with Grandfather in the Pine Barrens of New Jersey, learning the way of the scout—how to move silently through the forest, how to survive in any condition with nothing but the natural earth around him. As an adult, Tom dedicated himself to teaching others these skills.

Tom's outdoor classrooms and primitive-skills curriculum were a far cry from the polished yoga studios I was used to, and their elemental nature was just what I needed at that point in my life. But it was during the philosophy courses that I really understood why I was there.

Tom, through the wisdom of Grandfather, teaches what I can only describe as yoga. He teaches about the "spirit that runs through all things." He teaches about the duality of human nature and that balancing the physical with the spiritual can bring you to oneness. He teaches about the shaman path of walking between the worlds. And he teaches a form of meditation that blew my mind! It was almost an exact version of the yoga nidra meditation that Rod Stryker teaches. It opened my mind in a different way to the power we have if we can only learn how to tap into it, whether you're a yogi or a mountain man.

Grandfather was not a fan of sitting meditation. As a warrior, he needed to be in the clear and open mind of meditation while he was actively engaged with the physical world. He often didn't have the luxury of being able to sit still with his eyes closed. He used a form of meditation called wide-angle vision, which is when you relax and open your focus to your peripheral vision as you walk. It is one of the tools the scout uses to keep the mind as open as the world around him, always on high alert at the same time as being deeply relaxed. It served as an entry point to the walking meditations that he taught Tom and that Tom then taught to us, his students. Wide-angle vision is the window to the unconscious mind and to the spirit. It is in the unconscious mind that our huge potential lies, and the way to reach it is through meditation.

You already know how the power of visualization can help you begin to work with underlying forces and energy. In a lecture called "The Metamorphosis of Power," Tom teaches that we need to balance control of our visualization with the vividness of it. In most visualizations you are the audience; it is two-dimensional. To really access the power of visualization, you want to step into the movie instead of watching it. And you do this by *envisioning*.

When you envision something, you add emotion and feeling. Tom says your envisioning must be *packed* with emotion and feeling. You must become *empassioned* about what you are visioning, what you are trying to manifest. It isn't enough to see yourself with the new girlfriend, or winning that award, or living in the new house. You must feel yourself there. What is the setting? Can you feel the wind on your skin, your hair blowing around, the powerful overhead lights? What does it smell like? Is something baking in the kitchen? Did someone bring you flowers, and the scent is delicious? What are you wearing? Is it too tight? Is the fabric silky soft or itchy? Is it cold out? Are you sweating? Can you feel the sweat running down your body?

As you start to work with your desires and what you want to truly manifest, these tools will help you bring it to life. As Grandfather said, "Whatever is spiritually manifest becomes physically manifest provided it is empowered."

The Hunting Warrior: Manifesting Your Desires

Warrior energy is one that is often challenging to talk about in yoga classes. How can we square the yogic emphasis on nonviolence with the warrior?

"The Buddhist tradition defines the Warrior as 'one who has the courage to know oneself.' . . . [T]he Tibetan definition of a 'warrior' is 'one who faces one's own fear.' . . . [T]hey both define the Warrior path as inside your own being," says conflict resolution pioneer and author Danaan Parry in *Warriors of the Heart.*

I've spent a lot of time contemplating these definitions of a warrior, doing the practices in Parry's book, as well as practicing martial arts and the more traditional warrior arts of shooting, both bow and arrows and guns. Many people talk about the warrior mind as being fierce and fighting for whatever it is you believe in. Some people talk about the peaceful warrior, withdrawing from confrontation, in the vein of Gandhi and Martin Luther King, Jr. Some view warriors as fiercely devoted to achieving their goals in a heart-centered way.

I was intensely curious as to why there would be three warrior poses in yoga. Most yoga poses are named for animals (lion, dolphin, eagle, peacock) or nature (tree, mountain, half moon) or simple body positions (intense side stretch, side arm balance). Why three poses with the name *warrior?* Why not just call it extended bent-knee pose?

As an avid archer, I couldn't help but see the warrior poses as a sequence of archery moves: reaching for your arrow, nocking the arrow on the bow, pulling back the bowstring, releasing the arrow, and resting in the stillness of non-movement immediately after release, so the arrow flies true. I started to do my warrior poses as an archer. I also wanted to introduce a hunting aspect to the poses. I wasn't necessarily hunting for prey, but what was I shooting my arrow *at?* What was I aiming for in my life? And *how* was I doing it? Was I focused, quiet, intense, and certain? Or was I flailing around, reaching for everything, hoping I'd hit the mark?

When I brought this deeper intention to the poses, of shooting my arrow to a definite target, they felt infused with so much meaning that I enjoyed the intensity of warrior II instead of wondering when I could straighten my front leg. If you've ever sat in the forest waiting for a wild animal, you know the incredible patience and stillness required. If you move quickly or suddenly, you are immediately seen, and the animal will dash away. The skills required to be a warrior are patience, stillness, calm and steadiness, and then, the ability to act powerfully in an instant. Shoot the photograph before the bear leaves; fire your gun or arrow before the deer runs away. Immediately act on that once-in-a-lifetime chance that, after all your hard work, has suddenly presented itself. This, in my opinion, is the path of the warrior. And the following Three-Warrior Vinyasa is how to prepare for it.

Practice of the Week: The Three-Warrior Vinyasa

Through this series of poses, "the target" is what you're aiming for—what you want to manifest in your life. If it's a new job, see yourself in your office, or on the stage, or at the computer—whatever the job setting is. See and feel, *empower*, the specifics of the situation: What does the space look like? Who's around you? How do you feel here? Are you nervous, happy, content, excited, overwhelmed? Apply the tool of envisioning to your visualization, and you are strengthening your ability to experience the reality you want to exist.

Stand in tadasana. Step the left foot back as far as you easily can and turn the toes out 30 degrees. Bend the front knee. Both hips are still reaching to face forward. This is warrior I.

Start with your hands in front of your heart in triple warmer/heart mudra, then extend them, palms together, straight out in front of you. Now take the left hand, sweep it overhead, and cross it up, over, and behind your head to your right shoulder and squeeze the top of the shoulder; this is a triple warmer release. If you can't quite reach the shoulder, you can mime pulling an arrow out of the quiver at your back (figure 29), which establishes the ever-important crossover pattern in your body's energies.

Next extend both arms straight in front of you again and bring your hands together, palm touching palm (figure 30). With this position, you are nocking the arrow, or positioning it on your bowstring. Hold here, ground through your feet, see your target, and breathe three to five breaths, establishing a stillness and quiet inside.

Now come into warrior II. Lightly slide the left foot slightly farther back. Inching back the left foot establishes a stabler base from which to shoot your visualized arrow. It is also the position you need to hold as you're waiting for your target to come into position. Shift the hips so they are open and both facing left. The feet are about three feet apart. Anchor through the outside edge of the back foot. Deeply bend the front knee so it is going toward a 90-degree angle, making sure the knee is directly over the ankle. Make sure the torso is directly over the lower body; don't lean the upper body over the front leg as if you're reaching for something. Keep the weight evenly anchored over both feet. Note that this is a slightly narrower warrior II stance than typical.

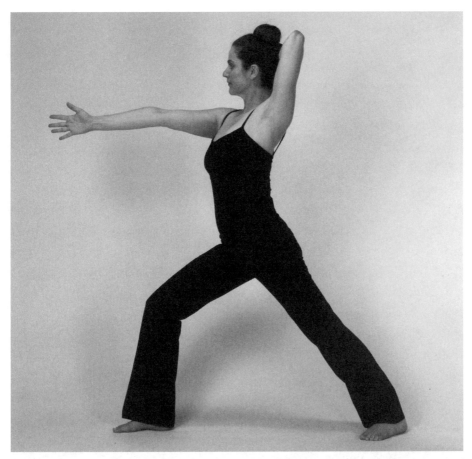

FIGURE 29   The Three-Warrior Vinyasa: warrior I, taking arrow from quiver, reinforcing the crossover

At the same time you are moving the feet and opening the hips, start to pull the bowstring back: slide the left hand along the inside of your extended right hand and arm across your body, until your open left hand rests above your heart with your thumb on the first point of lung meridian. (See figure 31.) This is warrior II. Stay here, sink into the pose, and breathe three to five breaths.

Now that your bow is drawn, take your left hand and tap along the temporal bone around your ear. Tap lightly on your skull from the temple, traveling behind the ear as if you were smoothing back your hair, front to back, three times. The temporal tap is an ancient technique that was used for pain control in TCM. It helps to calm triple warmer, as it lies directly on the triple warmer meridian and is moving against the natural flow of triple warmer. It helps to suspend sensory stimulation, making it easier for the brain to receive a new,

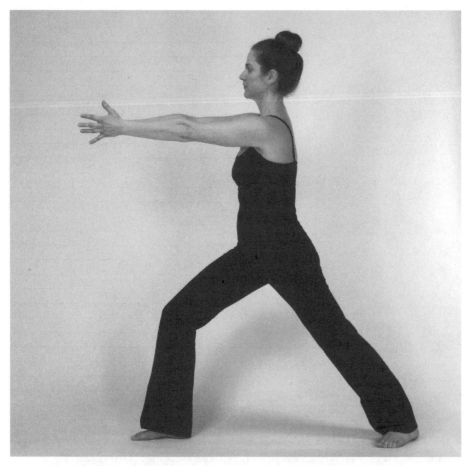

FIGURE 30   The Three-Warrior Vinyasa: warrior I, nocking the arrow on the bow

more directed form of input. The subconscious mind processes twenty million environmental stimuli per second. The conscious mind processes forty environmental stimuli per second. Using the temporal tap helps to interrupt the input of external stimuli, so the vision of your target, what you're trying to manifest, can enter the subconscious without the distraction of twenty million other stimuli.

Your right arm is still extended in front of you, holding the bow. Continue to breathe smoothly and steadily.

Once you have seen and felt and tapped in your target clearly, release the arrow, which launches you forward into warrior III. Your whole body follows the flying arrow, like the arm following the throw after the baseball has left the hand. (See figure 32.) But it is a slow movement. Look at your target as you

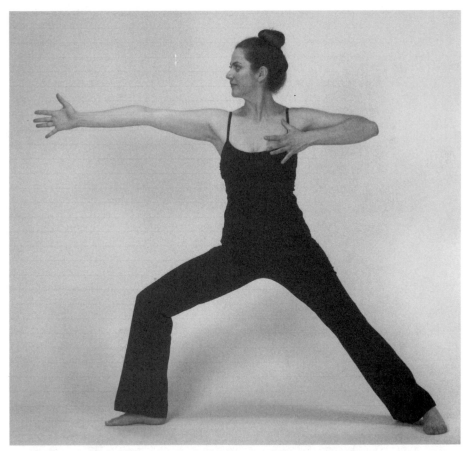

FIGURE 31   The Three-Warrior Vinyasa: transition from warrior I to warrior II; note that warrior II stance is narrower than usual

release your arrow and the left arm comes forward to meet the right in front of you. The left leg lifts up in the air behind you, hip and toe pointing down, to stabilize the pose. This movement happens slowly and deliberately; it is not a rush to get there. The steady, equal breath helps to keep your balance and focus. Your standing leg is strong and straight, with a slight microbend at the knee (figure 33).

After three to five breaths, during which you see yourself and your target merge into manifestation, step down lightly, back into warrior I, where you'll pull another arrow and begin the series again. After shooting two or three more arrows, come back to tadasana and switch sides.

Energy System of the Week: The Electrics

One of the most elegant systems in energy medicine, and the only system that can be measured with outside instruments, is the electrics, or the electrical

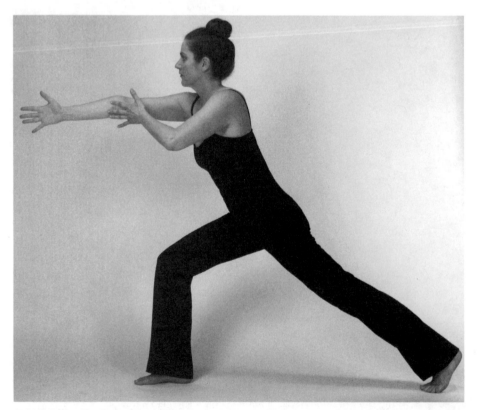

FIGURE 32   The Three-Warrior Vinyasa: transition from warrior II to III, releasing the arrow

system. All the other energy systems interact with the electric system. Every cell in the body has positive and negative charges within it, and the distribution of those charges causes the cells to vibrate. This vibration is electrical in nature. The energy systems have either electrical energies or electromagnetic energies, which are measurable fields. In *Introduction to Electrics,* Donna Eden, David Feinstein, PhD, and Vicki Matthews, ND, explain:

> The movement of electrically charged ions at the cellular level is the
> basic building block in the complex electromagnetic workings of
> your "body electric." Every muscle you move, every thought you
> think, every morsel of food you digest, involves electrical activity.
> Your feelings, memories, and thoughts are coded in patterns of
> tiny electrical impulses. Electrical fields help regulate tissue growth
> in the fetus and promote tissue regeneration in adults. Electrics
> relate to the heart, as it is the strongest electrical generator in the

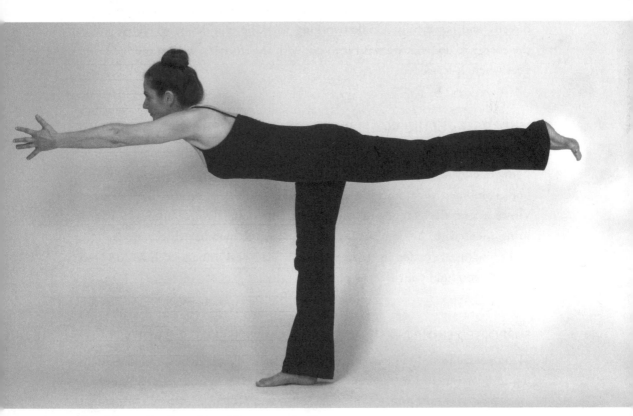

FIGURE 33   **The Three-Warrior Vinyasa: warrior III**

body. The heart makes hormones, has its own nervous system, and regulates your rhythm. It creates an alchemy of healing forces, assisting your immune system in keeping you well. The Electrics assist the heart in flowing these powerful hormones, thoughts, and feelings to the rest of the body.

Generally, work with the electrics is most efficient and powerful when done with a partner. The introduction of another person's energy field helps you to access your electrics. But you can hold your own electric points as well and still have a powerful, if subtler, effect on this system.

There are points on the body through which you can tap directly into the electric system, similar to the way the outlets in your house tap into your home's electrical wiring. Through these points, you can either direct electric energy to specific parts of the body or hold points that activate the natural electric intelligence of the body, which will go to work where needed. The main electric points, which we'll hold in two poses this week, hook us into this powerful energy field in order to affect the heart and the nervous system, subtly, but also directly and powerfully. Unlike working with the meridians, where we guide the energy to do what we want it to do, with the electrics, we just tap in, and it goes where it is needed.

More Poses of the Week: Restorative Inversions with Electric Holds

In my Energy Medicine Yoga classes, I regularly offer my students two inversions, both combined with powerful electric holds. After you do the Three-Warrior Vinyasa, take the potency of your target (the desires you're aiming for) and bring them with you during these two poses. Remember that your feelings and thoughts are coded in "patterns of tiny electrical impulses." Envision your desire as you hold your electric points.

SUPPORTED SHOULDERSTAND (*SIRSASANA*) WITH ELECTRIC HOLD

Many people love shoulderstand, and it has incredible benefits, including helping to flush out and strengthen the thyroid and parathyroid glands. But there are people who can't practice this pose because of neck or back issues, glaucoma, chronic headaches, or other contraindications. During regular shoulderstand, it is important to use props correctly. But often people don't know how to correctly use their props, or they choose not to, only to find later on that they've damaged their vertebrae. This modified version of the pose gives you all the benefits of the regular pose, with none of the dangers.

Have a block handy. Lie down on your back with your knees bent and your feet flat on the floor. Lift the hips off the floor and bring the block under the low back. For beginners, I recommend using the shortest height of the block with the widest expanse on the body. More-advanced practitioners can use the highest height of the block. Release your hips down onto the block. It should

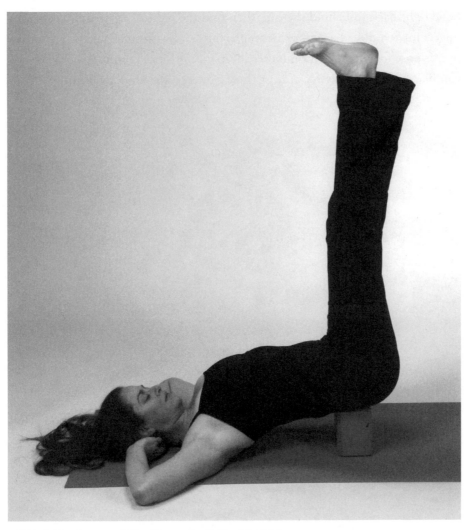

FIGURE 34   Supported Shoulderstand with Electric Hold

be located at your sacrum, and most of your bum should be off the block. This position should feel extremely comfortable, so adjust it until this is so.

Now lift both legs straight up in the air so they are at a 90-degree angle to the floor. If you can keep your legs straight, do so, and if you can keep your feet flexed, do this, too.

Bend your elbows and bring your hands behind your head to the occipital bone, where your head connects to the neck. In the very center, there is a deep hollow bordered by two ropy tendons. Move the first two fingers from each hand over these tendons to the slight hollow on either side. These are your main electric points. (See figures 34 and 35.)

First, deeply massage these points. You can also massage along this entire bone right back to behind the ear. Then find the hollows again and press your fingers in. You don't have to press deeply, but hold with some pressure. Remain in this pose for three to five minutes, deeply breathing. (You can stay longer, if you like, but try to stay for at least three minutes, the amount of time it takes

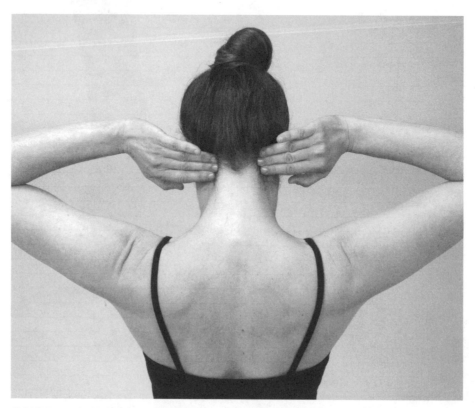

FIGURE 35   Location of the electric points

for the blood in the extremities to return to the heart for oxygenation.) You may feel your fingers start to buzz or grow hot. The two points may start to pulse together, like the meridian acupressure points. This is the electrical system waking up, responding to your input of energy and starting to cycle it through the body.

To release the hands, press into the hollows again and massage deeply, as if you are now unplugging your fingers, then smooth the hands outward.

Bend the knees and put the feet flat on the floor. Lift the hips and remove the block. Let the hips come back to the floor and let the knees soften toward each other to release the back. You can also bring the knees into the armpits, gently folding the back in while still lengthening the spine by pressing the buttocks toward the floor.

LEGS UP THE WALL (*VIPARITA KARANI*) WITH ELECTRIC HOLD

This pose is similar to supported shoulderstand, but you use the wall to help support the legs, turning this pose into a deep relaxation and restorative pose. Viparita karani, or legs up the wall pose, is an inversion that can be practiced when you are menstruating, unlike other inverted poses. If you are menstruating, do not use a block to elevate the hips, but keep them on the floor. This pose allows the venous blood returning to the heart to make the trip more easily, as the venous blood system does not have its own pump. This pose is also good for helping varicose veins or swollen ankles.

Lie on the floor on your side, with your butt at the edge of a wall. Slowly roll over onto your back and extend your legs up the wall, inching your hips as close to the wall as possible. You may want to experiment with putting folded blankets or a folded mat under your hips for utmost comfort. You can also bring a block to the edge of the wall and put it under your sacrum to elevate your hips. You'll be holding this pose for up to ten minutes, so it's a good idea to be as comfortable as possible.

Once you are comfortable, bring your hands behind your head, with your elbows out to the sides. Put your thumbs in the two hollows on either side of the thick, corded muscle at the back of your neck, right at the junction of your neck and your head into the main electric points. (You can experiment with what feels more comfortable, the thumbs in the electric points, or the fingers, as described above.) With your thumbs in the electrics, interlace your fingers and rest your head in your hands. Just as you felt with the neurovascular points and

the acupressure points, you will soon feel a slight pulsing and then a synchroniz-
ing of the pulses. As you hold here longer, you may also feel heat—quite a lot
of heat—or buzzing, as if your hands are falling asleep. You can stay here anywhere from three to ten minutes. This is also a great pose for helping to reboot
your energy when you're having that midday lag.

When you are ready to come out of the pose, release your thumbs from the
electric points by pressing in and twisting them slightly, to disengage the electrical current. Then bend your knees, slide your feet down the wall, and roll over
onto your right side. Rest for several moments here, letting the energy of the
pose settle into the body.

Tip: If you do these poses right after the Three-Warrior Vinyasa, you can
use the opportunity to continue visualizing what it is you want to manifest, as
you're holding the electric points. This helps to synthesize your thoughts into
their electrical charge.

Chakras and Shock Points

This week you learn how to release the energy of shock from the body and how to work with the chakras. Donna says that if you have only one opportunity to work with an energy-medicine client, do a chakra session. The chakras are that powerful. They are the hard drives of the information that makes us who we are. Working with the chakras can bring some of the deepest healing possible. Starting to release present or past shock from the body can help as we access the deeper information stored in the chakras.

Shock-Point Release

Shock can happen to the body quickly and without warning and be triggered by myriad events. Even perceived events can put us into shock. We can also have the energy of old shock still residing in the body. If a shock is severe enough, it can disrupt the basic systems that deliver the cellular needs of glucose and oxygen to the body, causing the body to start to shut down.

Nature knows how to release excess energy, as we see in a volcanic explosion, shifting tectonic plates in the earth, or flooding. We can see it in a dog who shakes his body after a harrowing encounter, or a deer, quivering all over to release excess energy after being chased. Releasing shock is something we humans need to learn. If we don't shake off this energy, that shaking will happen internally, working against our natural stillness, and disrupt our biological functions. Using breath and movement can help to clear disturbing energy so the body remembers balance. We simply need to help it on its way.

Working with what are known as the shock points can help to balance the sympathetic and parasympathetic nervous systems, as well as help to balance triple warmer and spleen meridians, all systems that get thrown off with shock.

When I teach this protocol, I pass out small semiprecious stones to my students. You can choose a stone that has a particular power to it that resonates with you.

First stand in tadasana and begin to pound your heels on the ground. Pound back and forth, trying to create as much force as you can. Keep weight on your toes, and bend the knees to pound the heels. Soon, the whole body will be shaking as you're drumming your heels back and forth on the ground. Let the body shake and tremble and release excess energy. You can do this for up to a full minute or two. Slowly bring yourself back to stillness and then stand there, breathing deeply, and feel the continued release of energy.

Now take the small stone and place it under one of your heels. You're going to roll the heel around on the stone, standing and pressing into the stone at different points under the heel. The main shock point is in the center, at the fleshiest part of the heel, and there are similar points in line with that closer to the center of the foot and closer to the heel. When you find a point that is particularly sore, spend a bit more time here. Once you find a shock point, pressing it should feel good and relieve your pain. You can spend as much time as you like on the first heel and then switch the stone to the other heel, or take two stones and do both heels at the same time. You'll feel a natural internal impulse to stop this practice when the body has released enough.

You can do this release as part of the Wake Up or before you start the sun salutations. For more on releasing trauma and shock, see the appendix.

Energy System of the Week: The Chakras

For anyone who has studied yoga, the chakras will be the most familiar of the energy systems.

The Sanskrit word *chakra* means "wheel," and the chakras are seen as wheels of energy that connect down into the body at the spine. The seven major chakras are situated along the spine, and there are many smaller chakras found throughout the body, including in the palms of the hands and the soles of the feet.

Each chakra consists of both an outward- and an inward-moving spiral. These two opposing spirals serve to bring energy and information both into and out of the body. Each chakra also has seven layers, which hold different kinds of information, from the mundane to the exalted and everything in between. The densest layer of a chakra is closest to the spine, and the least dense is farthest from the body. Donna Eden sees the layers connecting to each other with small figure-eight patterns that look like a sleeting rainfall. These eights help move energy and information between the layers.

The chakra system is basically the hard drive of the body's energetic systems, holding every experience and all our past and present information. The chakras also feed energy to the meridians and the organs found in their vicinity. The chakra system is closely related to the endocrine system; each chakra works with the endocrine glands in its realm. Each chakra also carries specific energies:

> The root chakra, *muladhara*, is located at the base of the spine
> and carries energies related to family, tribe, and security.
> The second chakra, *svadhisthana*, is located in the lower
> abdomen, between the belly button and the pubic bone, and
> carries energies of creativity, innocence, joy, and sexuality.
> The third chakra, *manipura*, is located at the solar plexus and
> carries the energy of ego, our personal identities, and our sense
> of power in ourselves and in the world.
> The fourth chakra, *anahata*, is located in the heart center and carries
> the energy of love—our ability both to receive and to give love.
> The fifth chakra, *vishuddha*, is located in the throat and carries
> the energy of communication and expression. This chakra
> also carries a pathway of energy for each of the other chakras,
> deciding, as energetic information comes into the body, in
> which chakra it belongs.
> The sixth chakra, *ajna*, is located at the third eye, between the
> eyebrows, and carries the energies of intuition, insight, and
> vision, and our connection to our own inner world.
> The seventh chakra, *sahasrara*, is located at the crown and carries
> the energies of our connection to the larger world and to the
> cosmos or the divine.

In yoga, all of the asanas, or postures, work to shift the energy of one or more chakras, and you can easily design an Energy Medicine Yoga practice to work specifically with chakra energies. As you learn the attributes of the chakras, you can see where your particular weaknesses lie and learn to strengthen them. For example, you can see where you may be weak physically, recognize if you are also lacking strength in those chakras' energies, and design your practice to strengthen them. Maybe your hips are always sore or tight. This would be related to the first chakra, and you could add more hip openers as well as work with the circulation-sex meridian neurolymphatic points to help release tension here. Conversely, you may have difficulty expressing yourself, feeling like you never say what you need or that you're never heard when you express your concerns. These symptoms are related to weakness in the throat chakra, and you might add this week's fish pose with chakra clearing to try to bring more energy and attention there.

Practices of the Week: Chakra-Clearing and -Balancing Sequence

The following two poses introduce the chakras into the practice of Energy Medicine Yoga. The first, fish pose with chakra clearing, helps open up the fifth chakra, which is not only the chakra governing our communication abilities, but also the chakra facilitating communication between all the other chakras. It is command central. By working with the chakras via the fifth chakra specifically, you can start to actually feel, through soreness in the channels in the throat, which other chakras may need more energy or support.

The second pose, a chakra-enhancing savasana, allows you to give the chakras in need that extra attention, as well as to attend to the health and vitality of all the chakras.

FISH POSE (*MATSYASANA*) WITH CHAKRA CLEARING

Donna sees the fifth chakra, located in the throat, as markedly different from the others. Instead of being a round swirl of energy, it is laid out along the neck in channels like the pipes of a pipe organ. Each chakra has a correlating pathway through the throat chakra, and each chakra transmits and translates its information and energy through this chakra of communication. The throat chakra is like the conductor of an orchestra, harmonizing information between the lower chakras and the chakras in the head. The throat chakra also decides which chakra to send incoming energetic information to for storage. Many people consider the heart chakra, the fourth, to be the connection point between the upper and lower chakras, but Donna sees this connection happening clearly in the throat chakra. By massaging and opening the throat in the following pose, you are helping to open and clear every chakra. Notice which areas may be sore, as this soreness could point you to a chakra imbalance that you can then work to correct with other practices.

Lie on your back with yours arms by your sides. Put your weight on your elbows and come to sit up halfway. Lift the heart center and slowly allow the head to move backward, creating a deep upper-body backbend. Slowly move the elbows along the floor, lowering the head until the crown is on the floor. Balance here, with the crown of the head, the buttocks, and the legs supporting the pose. You can also have weight in the elbows. If you want, you can bring the arms up and overhead with the palms touching. This position can be very hard on the cervical vertebrae. If you have any issues with your neck, head, or throat, modify this pose by keeping the weight fully on your elbows and/or letting the head hang free, not touching the floor. You can also put a bolster under the upper back so the head and neck are supported but still allowed to open and flex.

This pose creates a deep stretch at the throat, upper shoulders, and back and helps strengthen the thyroid and parathyroid glands, which are located at the base of the throat. It is also deeply oxygenating, opening the upper lungs. If you are comfortable here and are not resting weight on your elbows, you'll stay in this position while doing the chakra clearing. If the pose is already intense enough, release from fish pose as described at the end of these directions and then clear the chakras.

For clearing the chakras, bring the fingertips of both hands to the center of your throat. Smooth the fingers of one hand up and the fingers of the other hand down, with gentle pressure, along the centerline of the throat. (See figure 36.)

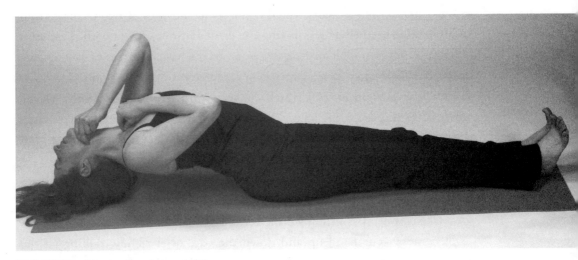

FIGURE 36   Clearing the chakras in fish pose

Move your fingers one inch to the right, keeping them level with the Adam's apple, and smooth the fingers of one hand up toward the jaw, and smooth the fingers of the other hand down toward the collarbone. Move your fingers another inch to the right and again smooth up and down. Move to the right one more inch, and you should be almost in line with your ear. Smooth up and down one last time.

Come back to the centerline, at the level of the Adam's apple, and smooth up and down again. Now move the fingers one inch to the left. Smooth up and down. Move another inch left, smooth up and down. Move the last inch to the left, almost to the ear, and smooth the last channel.

The centerline of the throat corresponds to the seventh chakra. Moving to the right, you are working the yang chakras, coming to the first, the third, and then the fifth, which is almost in line with your ear. Moving from the center to the left are the yin chakras; from center, you come to the second, then the fourth, and then the sixth chakra, almost in line with the left ear.

To come out of fish pose, bring your elbows back to the ground if you've lifted your arms, and put your weight on them. Slowly lift your head and then slowly lower your upper back and neck, making sure there's no strain in the neck. Relax here for several moments. If you did not do the chakra clearing in the full pose, do so now. Notice if there are any tender chakra columns. You'll work with those that stood out during the following version of savasana.

SAVASANA WITH CHAKRA LINK

In this variation on savasana, you'll connect the energies of two chakras. Your hands act like jumper cables, mixing the energy of one chakra with the energy of another. You can look at the description of the basic energies of each chakra earlier in this chapter to see which two energies you'd like to connect. Maybe you already have an idea of which chakras you'd like to work with. Maybe during the fish pose with chakra clearing you felt that two of the chakra channels were particularly sore. Or maybe you'll simply let the intuition of your hands find the two chakras that would benefit the most from connecting.

Lie in savasana, with your legs slightly separated and rolled open in their sockets. Allow your jaw to relax, and relax the tongue. Relax the eyes in the eye sockets. Release any control over the breath.

First move your hand up and down the core of the body, linking all the chakras together with figure eights. Weave your hand in a figure-eight pattern over the first two chakras, then the second and third, then the third and fourth, and so on, until you've woven yourself right up the centerline of the body to your sixth and seventh chakras.

Next bring one hand to cover one chakra and the other to cover another chakra. Perhaps you want to link your creativity with your sense of personal power, so you'll link the second and third chakras. Trust yourself and surrender. You can use padding to help elevate your arms, which is useful for resting your hands on the higher chakras, so you can completely surrender.

You can stay with your hands on your two chosen chakras for the entire savasana or until you feel complete. Then release your arms by your sides, palms facing up, and continue to deepen your relaxation.

If, after connecting the chakras, you still feel that a particular chakra needs more attention, you can "spin" the chakra to help it release or bring in energy. Bring your hand over the chakra and make circles, first in a counterclockwise direction, for three minutes. Then make circles in a clockwise direction for three minutes. End by holding both hands over the chakra you just cleared, and visualize it being bathed in light.

Weaving It All Together

This week, I'll show you how to arrange all the practices from the previous seven weeks into a complete, comprehensive Energy Medicine Yoga practice. This practice serves well as a daily routine and is the ideal foundation for a longer, customized practice. Before I give you the template, I'll give you two more valuable practices to include.

Coming Back to the Head: Powerful Points and Disruptive Forces

The first of this week's practices makes use of the healing and calming power of holding the head. All of the primary senses are in the head; the way we interact with the world starts here. All those bumps and knobs on your head are map points that help you find the many powerful points on the head—neurovascular reflex points, meridian starting and end points, electric points, and the power point itself, which is on the governing meridian. (The power point facilitates communication between the head and the body and helps to relax the body, as well as to increase psychic abilities.) Massaging or holding these different points can help relieve and release tension and built-up emotion, as well as help to dissipate trauma.

Any time you are in a yoga pose and can release the head into the hands, do it! Forward bends are the prime example of poses that allow you to release your head—in other words, to stop using the muscles in your neck to support it. When you are in a forward-bending pose, you can use a yoga block or a bolster to allow the head and neck to be supported and relax completely. If it's possible, release your head into your hands, allowing your hands and fingers to touch, massage, and/or hold points on your skull.

Also on the head are many points where energies called disruptive forces can enter the body. The disruptive forces are environmental energies that can come in and wreak havoc with the body's energies. These energies—wind, heat, damp, dry, and cold—can overwhelm the triple warmer response and make it hard to understand why things aren't going well in the body. But there is also a flip side to these energies. Sometimes it's good for us to be disrupted. Some of the best things in our lives come to us in crazy, unplanned ways. And if we are closed to them, we'll miss out.

We don't want to barricade the doors against these energies; instead we want to keep ourselves balanced so we can not only withstand them, but also utilize them. Senior Eden Energy Medicine teacher Dr. Sara Allen teaches about the disruptive forces using the wonderful metaphor of "keeping our screens clean." If we keep these points clear, the five environmental energies can flow into us, bringing change, but have an exit as well. Since many of these screen points are located on the head, doing the Crown Pull (see week 1) is helpful, as are massaging, holding, and releasing the head into the hands as noted above. Also helpful is a practice I developed called Bean with Head Heal.

Practices of the Week: Healing and Calming, the End of Your Practice

Here are two final practices to include in your basic Energy Medicine Yoga routine. The first brings us back to the powerful points on the skull, which we worked with in week 1. The second draws the power of visualization into the close of any yoga practice: savasana.

BEAN WITH HEAD HEAL

We start in child's pose and eventually lean forward onto the elbows. This "growing out" of the child always reminds me of a sprouting bean—hence, the name Bean with Head Heal.

Start in child's pose. Bring your hands behind your head and massage all along the occipital ridge, all the way to the backs of the ears. Spend some extra time at the hollow right behind your ear lobe; this is triple warmer 17, the Shielding Wind entrance points—one of the screens we want to keep clean.

Next, massage deeply several times around the ear, from the top of the ear around to the lobe. Go right against the fold of the ear and all the way out to the temporal bone, the hard, bony ridge that follows the ear.

Bring your elbows forward and prop your head on your hands. The heels of the hands should be on the cheekbone, pressing into the stomach meridian points beneath the eyes, as well as other points that affect the nasal cavity. The thumbs rest lightly above the ears near the temples; these are triple warmer neurovascular points, and holding them is very calming. The palms of the hands cover the eyes, which helps to calm and sooth the optic nerve. (See figure 37.) Almost 80 percent of the tension in the human body resides in the eyes, and if you can relieve some of this tension, you can go a long way toward releasing tension in the body. Palming (covering the eyes with the palms) is one way to do this. The fingers extend up on the forehead into the hairline. They are covering the frontal neurovascular points, the main points in the neurovascular system, as well as the liver neurovasculars, which enhances the body's ability to metabolize hormones.

While you're holding your head in this position, experiment with exactly where the elbows should be placed in relation to the head and neck to maximize the relaxation of the neck. Let the jaw go completely, allowing the lower jawbone to fall forward. In this pose, you can really start to feel the architecture of your bones.

Stay as long as you like, continuing to breathe deeply and to surrender. If emotions come up, just stay with them, allowing the energy to move through. This is a powerful pose to start to transmute the energetic charge of intense emotions. (The appendix will also give you more tools for transmuting intense emotions.)

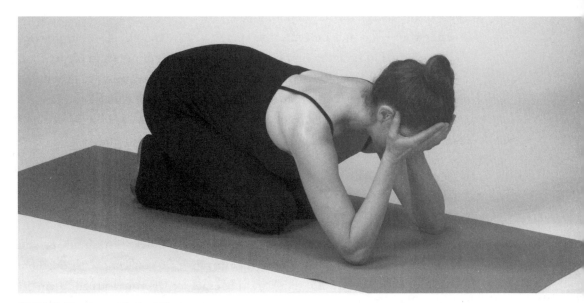

FIGURE 37   **Bean with Head Heal**

SAVASANA WITH ENERGY SYSTEM VISUALIZATION

Savasana is a wonderful time to practice visualizing the energy systems of the body, letting your mind's eye actually turn on and move these energies. Several teachers, including Donna Eden, teach how to move the energy with the mind. There are many tantra yoga techniques, as well, in which you visualize and move energy with your mind.

In your relaxation, you can see energy systems moving, activating, integrating. You can open up your chakras, making them spin both inwardly and outwardly. You can trace the flows of specific meridians. You can trace the flow of the radiant circuits, knit your aura, draw figure eights in the Celtic Weave—all while you are in this deeply resting, open state. Energy flows where attention goes.

There are many wonderful books with photos or drawings of what the energy systems look like, if you'd like some visual templates to start with. Donna has drawings in her book *Energy Medicine.* Energy medicine teacher Barbara Brennan has some wonderful illustrations in her books. The artist Alex Grey also creates incredible art based on the energetics of the body.

Savasana is a perfect time to tune in and follow the energies that are moving as a result of your practice. Feel where energy is moving, and how. Does it have a color? A sound? Follow it as it moves through the body. You may be following a particular flow of energy moving naturally up a meridian path or through a chakra. In this way, you start to develop the more refined senses and become aware of the energy that is animating your body.

After you've felt and moved some energy, release the visualization practice and spend time in savasana simply being, with the mind open and empty.

When you feel complete, anywhere from five to fifteen minutes depending on the length of your physical practice, slowly start to wake yourself up. Deepen your breath and move your hands and feet. Roll over onto your right side and take several deep breaths here. Then slowly begin to sit up.

Putting the Practices Together: Your Energy Medicine Yoga Practice

If you combine key practices and techniques from weeks 1 through 8, you will have an ideal Energy Medicine Yoga practice. If you choose to do them all together, you won't do them in the exact order you learned them in, because sometimes the concepts that lead to the poses need to come earlier in the teaching cycle than the physical poses come in the sequence. Intelligent sequencing, called *vinyasa krama,* helps us lay out a practice that follows the energy patterns of the body and helps us open the body up in an intelligent way.

We start, as always, waking the body up. Then we follow with standing poses, inversions, backbending poses, seated poses and twists, restorative inversions, and savasana.

The template on the following pages gives you the most important poses from the preceding seven weeks. If you do just the most powerful and necessary practices, the routine will take you twenty to forty minutes. You can adjust how much time you spend in the poses as you start to get the feedback from your body. Hooking up the meridians, for example, takes longer when you're just beginning to work with them, but soon you'll find them synching up more quickly, giving you more time for other things. That's the cumulative and empowering effect of Energy Medicine Yoga; the results are tangible and teaching you. The optional practices listed can be added into your practice or substituted for other techniques to give you more balance and variety.

Consistency and Dedication

I encourage you to dedicate a certain amount of time every day to an Energy Medicine Yoga practice, just as you dedicate a certain amount of time every day to brushing your teeth. You are dedicating time to yourself. Even if you are too busy to do the template practice, you can do many of the practices on their own at any time during your day. Even five minutes a day is a valuable piece of real estate and a potent gem to start with. Energy moves quickly, but deep patterns in the body need time and space to shift. Many of my students have found that using these techniques actually make them more efficient in the rest of their lives, allowing more time to practice, which then makes them more efficient and less stressed in the rest of their lives, providing a positive feedback loop for continued self-care.

ENERGY MEDICINE YOGA TEMPLATE

CHECK-IN: How do I feel at the start of my practice?

① THE WAKE UP (week 1, page 11)

    The Four Thumps

    The Cross Crawl

    The Zip Up

    The Hook Up

    Optional
- Head Massage, Crown Pull, Spinal Flush
- Cat Pose (chakravakasana) with mula bandha (week 3, page 60)
- Thread the Needle (sucirandhrasana) with Yang Bridge Flow (week 3, page 61)

② SQUAT WITH GAIT CLEARING (week 1, page 24)

③ HANG WITH GAIT CLEARING AND INTESTINE DETOX MASSAGE (week 1, page 26)

④ ENERGY MEDICINE YOGA SUN SALUTATION(S) (week 2, page 40)

    Optional
- Additional standing poses and inversions
- Three-Warrior Vinyasa (week 6, page 108)

⑤ FIVE-ELEMENTS SALUTATION (week 5, page 95)

⑥ DYNAMIC BRIDGE POSE (SETU BANDHA SARVANGASANA) WITH NEUROLYMPHATIC CLEARING (week 3, page 62)

    Optional
- Fish Pose (matsyasana) with Chakra Clearing (week 7, page 122)
- Additional backbends
- Slow Sit-Ups with the Triple Warmer–Spleen Hug (week 4, page 75)
- Additional seated poses and twists

(7) KIDNEY THREE-POINT POSE (week 4, page 78) or HEAD-TO-KNEE POSE
(JANU SIRSASANA) WITH SPLEEN STRENGTHENING (week 4, page 82)

Optional
- Cobbler's Pose (baddha konasana) with Gait Clearing (week 4, page 87)
- Child's Pose (balasana) with Spinal Flush (week 3, page 62)
- Bean with Head Heal (week 8, page 128)

(8) SUPPORTED SHOULDERSTAND WITH ELECTRIC HOLD (week 6, page 114) or
LEGS UP THE WALL (VIPARITA KARANI) WITH ELECTRIC HOLD (week 6, page 117)

Optional
- Eye yoga

(9) SAVASANA WITH CHAKRA LINK (week 7, page 124) or
SAVASANA WITH ENERGY SYSTEM VISUALIZATION (week 8, page 130)

Optional
- Pranayama practice — amount of time:
  Type: sama vritti, ujjayi, alternate nostril,
  mental alternate nostril, pure breath.
- Meditation practice — amount of time:

CHECK-IN: How do I feel after my practice?   Length of total practice:

What did I learn in today's practice?

What's Next?

When I first came out west at sixteen years old, I learned how to bushwhack—to walk off the designated trail and find a route on my own. Bushwhacking is an easy way to get lost and discombobulated, and it is a powerful way to learn how to read terrain and discover your own path through the wilderness.

In the same way, you can choose to leave the template and find your own way in your Energy Medicine Yoga practice. Part 1 has given you not only poses and practices, but also the tools and skills for listening to your body and its energies. As you've been doing the practices, you've been developing your ability to sense what is going on with your energy systems and how to shift them. So through your practice and your breath, you can discover what feels good. What opens up your body? What allows you to move through your emotions instead of holding onto them? What gives you that extra charge to get through your day? What helps you get through that stressful meeting? Follow your body and your energy, and you'll start to be able to answer the question "What next?" in every situation, not only on your mat, but in your life.

In part 2, there are many more poses that you can experiment with. You can fold them into the template, to start to really customize your Energy Medicine Yoga practice and make it uniquely your own, or you can add them to your regular yoga practice to get more bang for your buck.

Expanding and Customizing Your Energy Medicine Yoga Practice

The practices in part 2 will help you take your Energy Medicine Yoga routine deeper. If you are used to practicing yoga for an hour or longer, these poses will help you round out your routine. There are also some longer practice sequences. They are arranged by type so you can easily find, say, a standing pose or a backbend, to insert into your practice template.

As you've been working and learning the concepts from part 1, hopefully you've been tuning in to how you feel physically, mentally, and emotionally as you're practicing. This tuning-in will give you the feedback that will guide you to customize your practice. If you've been noticing points on the body that are sore, you'll spend extra time tapping and massaging them to get the stuck energy moving. If you've got lots of sore points, you'll spend more time working the neurolymphatic points in poses like bridge and hang. If you find that the chakra lines on the throat in fish pose are sore, you'll spend time working those chakra areas. You might add more twists if the first three chakras are in greater need, or more backbending if it's the upper chakras, or more inversions if it's the top two chakras. If you find areas of the body that feel closed off, you might work more with the vayus and the breath. If you've discovered that thumping, crossover techniques, and weaving figure eights on and around your body makes you feel more alert, you'll add more of those to your practice.

Keep in mind that less is more. In Eden Energy Medicine, we learn about the connectivity of the body's energy systems. The body-mind truly is holistic. There are frequently many systems or parts of systems that are out of balance. For example, it is not unusual for someone to have three, four, five, or more meridians that are under- or over-energized, throwing off all the meridians, as well as affecting other systems and the overall health of the client. But the body is beautifully orchestrated, and you don't need to spend the entire session correcting each of the disrupted meridians. Often, if you correct and work with one, it balances and strengthens all of them. And balancing and strengthening the meridians, in turn, balances and strengthens other energy systems. This elegance is at work in all we do. The body wants to find balance. This is its natural and most desired state. And it wants to find its balance in the most efficient way possible.

You don't need to practice Energy Medicine Yoga for hours (though you certainly can, and you'll feel great!). You need to find the areas or systems that are not working optimally and start to bring attention to them. And if you take the time to do a daily practice and keep all of the major systems of your body working well, you can keep the dance of living in a fine balance.

As you expand and customize your Energy Medicine Yoga practice, here are some important concepts to remember. They are a part of every Energy Medicine Yoga practice I do and teach. You've already learned them in part 1, though you may not have realized it.

> **Breathe!** Use a dynamic, full breath and connect breath to movement.
> Allow the body to be **easeful, steady, and calm.** This is the yogic concept of *Sthiram, Sukham, Asanam.*
> Work toward the **centerline,** bringing your awareness into the spine.
> **Shake off excess energy** from hands and body as you practice.
> **Cross and weave** as much as possible—a simple swipe from the shoulder to the opposite hip, or weaving your hands in crossover patterns as you transition into, out of, and through poses.
> **Hook up the central and governing meridians** several times during your practice.
> At the end of every practice, take a generous **savasana.** This is the time the body integrates and transforms. Don't skip this step!

Standing Poses

Crossing and Lifting Energies in the Core

The poses in this sequence all include simple techniques to help clear, organize, or calm the energy generated by the intensity and strength of standing poses.

SPINAL SUSPENSION TWIST

The spinal suspension twist helps to rejuvenate and energize you. It affects all the meridians and chakras by elongating and stretching the spine and opening the shoulder blades. It also helps to reinforce the crossover pattern.

Stand with your feet two to three feet apart, toes turned slightly outward. Lean forward and press your hands onto the tops of your thighs, above your knees. This pose is known as horse pose or goddess pose.

Drop your left shoulder forward, twisting your spine, and, using your arms as fulcrums, press out of your waist (figure 38). Take three long, deep breaths, inhaling through the nose and exhaling through the mouth. Switch sides.

FLYING-UP LOCK (UDDIYANA BANDHA)
WITH FIRE KRIYA (AGNISARA DHAUTI)

In the same leg position as the spinal suspension twist, center the body and lean over with your hands on your thighs. Exhale all your air out through the mouth, and while holding the air out of the body, draw the chin down and slightly in, applying jalandhara bandha. Then draw the internal organs in and up, applying uddiyana bandha. Finally, draw mula bandha up. Hold all of the bandhas as you hold the breath out.

When you feel the need to inhale again, release all three bandhas and, slowly and with ease, inhale. When you've completed your inhale, stand up.

It is important that you release the bandhas first, before inhaling and standing up, and that you don't hold the air out for so long that you need to gasp when you're ready to inhale. Be gentle, and go slowly.

Once you feel confident with this practice, you can try flapping the abdominal wall. Exhale all the breath out, apply the bandhas, and then pull in and push out the belly several times, creating a suction. The breath is held out during the entire time. Again, when you feel the need to inhale, release all of the bandhas first, and then gently inhale as you come to stand. This movement is known as the fire kriya. A kriya is a cleansing exercise, and this is one of the most powerful for helping the digestive fire, as well as toning and massaging the abdominal organs and the diaphragm. It also stimulates the five vayus, especially samana, with its main location in the abdomen.

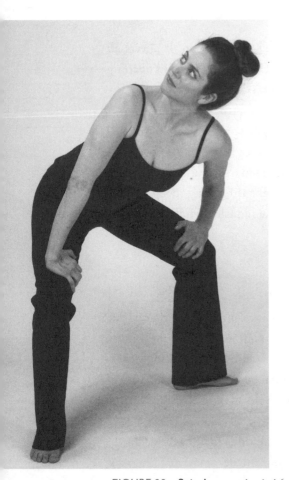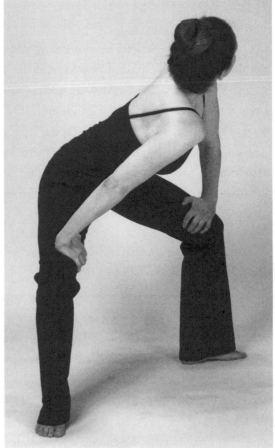

FIGURE 38   Spinal suspension twist

Doing the spinal suspension twist followed by uddiyana bandha and the fire kriya is deeply cleansing and detoxifying. This two-practice sequence helps to separate the lower body from the upper body, creating more awareness and demarcation in the core. It gives you more space into which to bring your attention for focused concentration and meditation if you choose to add these to the end of your physical practice.

Note: uddiyana bandha and the fire kriya are not to be practiced if you are menstruating or pregnant.

ILEOCECAL AND HOUSTON VALVES RESET

Directly after doing the previous two practices is the perfect time to reset these two most important valves in the body: the ileocecal and Houston valves. This can seem like a strange and esoteric practice, but it is easy and quick and can yield big results.

The ileocecal valve controls the flow of discarded waste, chemicals, and hormones from the small intestine to the large intestine. This valve is located on the right side of the body. Mirroring it, on the left, is the Houston valve, which is actually more of a bend in the colon than a true valve, but acts in a similar stopgap manner between the descending colon and the rectum.

As noted in the materials for class 1 of the Eden Energy Medicine Certification Program, "Donna talks frequently about the havoc these two valves can wreak in the body if they are out of synch, mimicking at least 27 serious illnesses. Resetting both valves together creates a symmetry between them. The rhythmic pulsing of these valves are [sic] also linked to all the other valves in the body, and so it is beneficial to them all if these two masters are reset. And this is easily done."

To reset these valves, put your hands on your low abdomen, with your pinky fingers resting on the inside edge of the hip bone, or the ileac crest (figure 39). As you inhale, press all your fingers with equal pressure into the body and smooth up several inches. Exhale, through the mouth, and shake off your hands. Do this three more times. Finally, start at the top of the swipe, inhale, and as you exhale, press your fingers into your body and smooth back down to the starting point.

Tree Pose (*Vriksasana*) with Triple Warmer/Heart Mudra to Warrior III (*Virabhadrasana* III)

Stand in tadasana and gently shift your weight to your left foot. Be sure that you don't collapse your hips, but try to keep the hip points balanced and level.

Bend your right knee and turn the knee out to the side, rotating the leg from the femur bone, not the hip. Bring the sole of the foot to the standing leg. If balancing is a challenge, you can keep the toes on the floor and the heel pressed against the left ankle. You can also use a wall for balance. If your balance is stable and you want to continue developing the pose, begin to slide the right foot up the leg, keeping the right knee bent and the right femur rotating outward. Draw the foot up as high as you like; just don't have the foot resting against the knee, as this is the weak point of the standing leg. You can use your

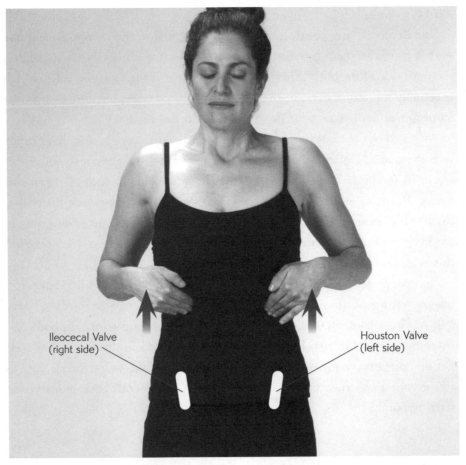

Ileocecal Valve
(right side)

Houston Valve
(left side)

FIGURE 39   Ileocecal and Houston valves

hands to reach down and bring the right foot all the way up into the groin, and if you're quite flexible, feel free to bring the foot into half lotus, as long as you can keep the foot there without holding it with your hand.

Draw the energy of the pose into the centerline of the body. Press the right foot into the left leg as much as you press the left leg into the right foot. Apply mula bandha to help increase the balance.

Now lift your hands up into triple warmer/heart mudra, with your thumbs in the heart center and the tips of your index fingers in the throat hollow. Allow your shoulder blades to deepen into the spine as well as sink down the spine. Also allow a slight opening in the front of the chest by pressing the chest up into your hands, as if you were opening up into the space between your hands. Activate this lift from the upper back, not from the lower rib cage. Find a point to focus on, at eye level, and breathe deeply.

If you want to develop the pose further, lift the arms up overhead, into dancing tree, and slowly drop the right elbow onto the lifted right knee and take a gentle side bend. Allow yourself to be playful here, and don't worry about falling out of the pose. Feel yourself as grounded as you are lifted.

When you come back to center, open both arms up overhead in a wide V. Lift up from the heart center and bring your gaze up to the sky. This is a pose called Heaven Rushing In, and in it you can gather inspirational energy from your "source," whatever you consider that source to be.

When you've allowed this energy to bathe you, come back to center and bring your hands back to the triple warmer/heart mudra.

From here, you can step out of the pose, or you can release the right foot from the left leg and bring it straight forward into extended hand-to-big-toe pose (*utthita hasta padangusthasana* C). Don't let the lifted leg push the torso back, but keep the body straight. Engage uddiyana bandha and jalandhara bandha to help maintain this intensely strengthening pose.

Now move the leg through center without letting it touch the floor and bring the leg straight back into warrior III (virabhadrasana III). Keep the hands in the triple warmer/heart mudra to help you keep the upper back from caving forward. Try to keep the extended right leg parallel to the floor. Breathe deeply three to five breaths.

Return to standing and step down, release your hands, and close your eyes. Allow yourself to feel the stability and strength of the tree.

Repeat the sequence on the other side.

Belt Flow to Side Twist (*Parivrtta Prasarita Padottanasana*)

Most of the energies of the body run up and down, like the meridians, and cross over, like the Celtic weave, or they have intricate patterns that they start in and then move off from, like the radiant circuits. There is only one energy, which also happens to be a radiant circuit, that runs horizontally through the body, at the waist. This is the belt flow. As explained in week 2, this energy flow helps connect and distribute the energies of the upper and lower body. It calms triple warmer and helps open the energy flow between the three warmers. It is also responsible for how grounded we are and how high we can reach. Think about the trunk of a tree: The roots descend below the earth deeply, and the branches reach up to the sky. If the roots are too shallow, the tree can't reach upward to its full potential. Helping us grow to our full potential is one of the jobs of the belt flow.

This flow is perfect to activate prior to doing twists, which initiate in the midsection. By activating the belt flow first, you assure that the twisting is done holistically and isn't separating your body, but is rather helping the body to integrate the up-down flow of energy. The belt flow runs through the body cavity and works with the diaphragm as well as the digestive organs. It helps to increase samana vayu. Unresolved feelings and emotions can get stuck in the belt flow, so working this region can help move and resolve emotions.

Stand in tadasana and reach both hands around to the left waist; you can even reach them behind the waist, if possible. With pressure, smooth both hands around the front of your waist across to the right side. Go back to the starting place, far on the left waist, and smooth the hands to the right again. Do this one more time and then smooth your hands down the outside of your right leg and off the right foot. Shake your hands off.

Repeat this movement on the other side, smoothing from the right waist to the left and ultimately off the left leg and foot.

Now separate your feet three feet apart, and keep your toes parallel. Open your arms up to shoulder height. Twist around and reach your left arm across the front of the body and down to the right leg, bending at the waist into this deep forward-bending twist. You can place your hand anywhere on the leg that feels comfortable—the knee, the ankle, the foot. If you're more flexible and the hand comes all the way down to the floor, put your hand down on the outside of your foot. Wherever your hand is, make sure you turn it so the fingertips are pointed backward.

Inhale, and return to standing. Do this dynamic preparation three times: inhale to start, exhale and reach across and down, inhale back to standing, and exhale. After the third breath, remain in the twist and breathe deeply.

Because of the position of the legs, the left hip will often swing widely forward to accommodate this twist. This may make you feel like you're deeper in the twist, but actually you are just turning the body. Instead, bring the hips back into alignment and keep them centered over the legs and allow the twist to come from the navel. Try to keep the hips equally balanced over the centerline as you twist from the core. To go deeper, extend your arms vertically—one down to the ground, the other stacked straight on top, so they form a straight up-and-down axis.

You may want to do another belt flow before you repeat the sequence on the other side.

Triangle Pose (*Trikonasana*) with SLK and Stomach Line Clear

In this pose you'll work with a potent merging of three points, as well as work a part of the stomach meridian called the stomach line.

From tadasana, separate your feet three feet apart. Turn the right toes 90 degrees to the right, and turn the left toes in slightly. Slightly tilt the hips back to the left and lean the right hand over into triangle pose (trikonasana). Lift the left arm straight up into the air.

Bring your right hand to the inside of your right calf, along the tibia bone. With your thumb, press in deeply along the back edge of the bone, where the muscle meets it. Deeply press into and smooth down the calf as far as you can go. (See figure 40.) Three meridians—kidney, spleen, and liver—all pass in and out of this zone. This is an area that is habitually sore and where the energies of these three meridians get stuck. Massaging down this area, against the flow of the meridians, helps to clear this stuck energy. If there are points that are particularly sore, work them more. (You have to keep the legs strong and active here while using your hand to massage these points. Be careful that you don't hang off the muscles or hyperextend the leg.)

You might find that your thumb drops right into a hollow halfway down the edge of the calf muscle, slightly out from where it meets the bone. This is the SLK point, a powerful convergence of these three yin meridians. It is guarded by the massive yang muscles of the calf. It is at this point that the yin energy decides if it's safe to move up into the body. Working this section of the leg, and especially the SLK point, helps to relax the yang muscles and meridians, led by triple warmer, and to tell the body it is safe for the yin energies to rise. The yin organs run the body, and without the yin energy to keep them strong, they are unable to do their endless, myriad tasks.

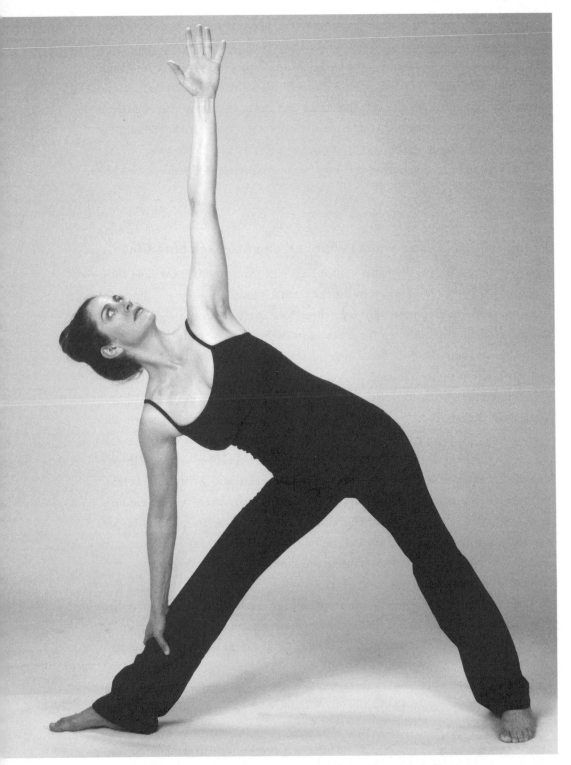

FIGURE 40   Triangle Pose (Trikonasana) with SLK and Stomach Line Clear

When you're done, move your fingers back up to the knee and then to the outside of the same calf bone. Smooth your fingers strongly down the outside of the bone where it meets the muscle. Here you are working the stomach line, or the bottom part of stomach meridian. This helps send energy down to the earth so you can pull kidney energy up. It also releases abdominal gas and helps with digestion. You can smooth this meridian a couple of times, from the knee down to the ankle. You cannot have a strong kidney 1 point if you don't have strong stomach chi, and deeply working this line helps to build stomach chi. You'll also move over stomach 36, which comes after the bend in the knee and is considered one of the most powerful acupressure points on the body.

After the meridian massage, remain in triangle pose for a few clearing breaths. Now extend the right arm up, parallel to the floor, and using the muscles of the side body, inhale back to stand.

Repeat on the other side.

VARIATION: LOW LUNGE WITH SLK AND STOMACH LINE CLEAR

You can also clear the SLK and stomach line in a low lunge. Step the left foot way back. Let the left knee come to the floor. Bend the right knee at a 90-degree angle; make sure the knee is right over the ankle and not leaning out or in. Lift the arms overhead (this is another great chance to weave the arms back and forth), then release the arms down and bring the hands to either side of the calf muscle where it connects to the bone. Smooth down the muscle, then spend some extra time on the SLK point. On the outside of the calf muscle, smooth down the stomach line (figure 41). Repeat on the other leg.

Wayne Cook Pose

The energy medicine practice called the Wayne Cook pose can keep you together when you're about to lose it. It was developed by Wayne Cook, a pioneering researcher of the body's energy fields. It is so powerful because it connects the back brain and the front brain—the primal brain and the modern brain—and thus links our ancestral fear impulses with our more developed reasoning faculties. It hooks up all the meridians and helps to integrate the body and mind so that you aren't working at cross-purposes from yourself, but are able to calmly see the situation you're in and your next step forward.

Eagle pose (*garudasana*) in yoga is nearly an exact execution of the Wayne Cook pose, and I believe it was used for similar purposes. Eagle pose is about soaring high and easefully above the situation at hand, while being able to see it all clearly laid out in front of you, just like an eagle able to see a tiny mouse a half mile below him in a field. It is also about deep integration, as the body is wrapped up as tightly as possible, while still maintaining stability; in other words, it integrates all the systems together into a coherent, grounded whole.

There are three options for this pose.

HIP STRETCH WAYNE COOK (CHAIR POSE VARIATION)

Stand in tadasana and gently shift your weight to your left foot. Balancing on the left leg, bring the right ankle to rest above the left knee, as if you were sitting in a chair. Then begin to bend the left leg (this is a modified chair pose). You're getting a deep thigh stretch in your outwardly rotated right thigh as you balance on your bent left leg.

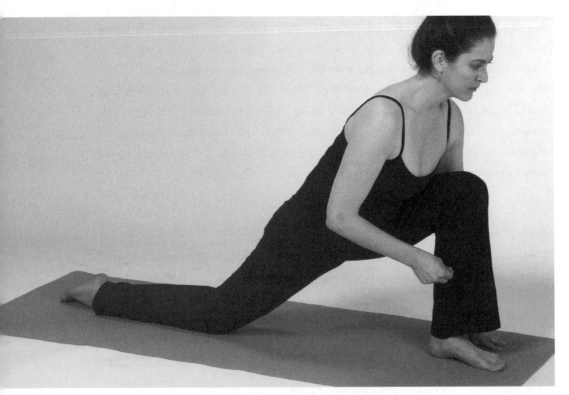

FIGURE 41   Low Lunge with SLK and Stomach Line Clear

Now hold the right ankle with your left hand, and take the right hand and wrap it around the ball of the right foot. (Notice that you're holding the foot and hands in a crossover pattern.) As you deeply stretch and balance here, pull your body slightly up and away from the bent leg on an inhale. Exhale through your mouth and relax back into the pose. (See figure 42.) Do this two more times.

Slowly unpretzel yourself, flying the limbs open, and switch sides. Now you'll be standing on the right leg, with bent knee, and crossing the left ankle over the right knee. Hold onto the left ankle with the right hand and the ball of the left foot with the left hand. Again, inhale, and pull the upper body away even as you sink into the legs. Exhale through your mouth and relax. Take two more breaths, and then release and stand up.

Inhale and circle your arms around overheard and bring your palms together. Bring your hands down to the level of your forehead, and place your thumbs in the center of your eyebrows, over your third eye. Inhale here, and as you exhale, smooth the thumbs apart on the forehead, spreading the skin.

Inhale again and now curl your fingers into the center of your forehead. Exhale and smooth them apart, spreading the skin. Release the arms and relax.

SCHOOLYARD HOOK UP

The second option for the Wayne Cook is called the Schoolyard Hook Up. If you have difficulty balancing or doing full eagle, or you want to teach this practice to kids, this version is the one for you.

Stand in tadasana and cross your right foot over your left, continuing to stand on both feet. Bring your hands straight out in

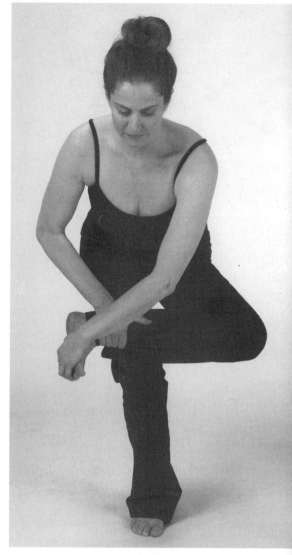

FIGURE 42   Hip Stretch Wayne Cook (chair pose variation)

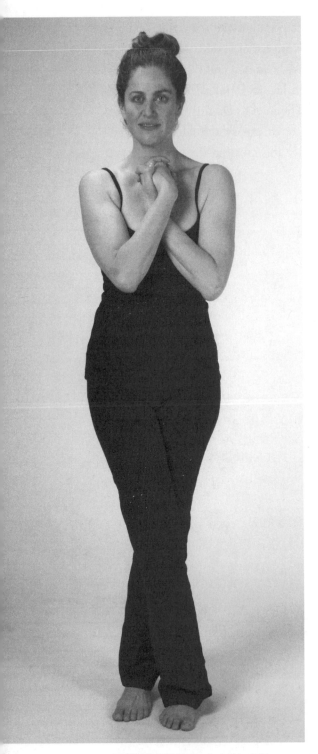

FIGURE 43   Schoolyard Hook Up,
a variation of the Wayne Cook pose

front of you, turn your palms away from you, thumbs facing down, and cross the left arm over the right. Bring the hands together, interlacing the fingers, and then scoop them up and under your chin. (See figure 43.) Take three deep breaths here.

Switch sides. Now the left foot will cross over in front of the right, and the right arm will cross over the top of the left. Interlace the fingers and scoop the arms up and under. Again, take three breaths.

Release both the feet and the hands. Again circle your arms up and overhead, and then bring them down and press the thumbs into the third eye. Inhale, and draw the thumbs apart, smoothing out the skin as you exhale. Then press the fingers into the center of the forehead and draw them apart, smoothing out the skin.

Tip: For the above two poses, try breathing in through your nose and out through your mouth. Then for full eagle, come back to yogic breathing, in and out through the nose.

FULL EAGLE

The third option is the full eagle pose. From tadasana, balance your weight on your left leg and bend the left knee. Cross the right knee over the left knee tightly, and if you can cross the right ankle behind the left ankle, do that as well.

The arms here are different from the second variation. This time you cross the left arm over the right, but keep the backs of the hands facing each other.

Then, if you can, cross the right arm up and over the forearm of the left arm to bring the palms of the hands together.

To deepen the pose, sink down in the legs, and bring the arms up, while keeping the shoulders down. Activating mula bandha will help you balance. Find a fixed point to look at, at eye level, to also help you balance. Take several breaths here and then switch sides.

Tip: Gazing at a fixed point is also a means of getting a feel for what it is in your life that you want to focus on and go after. Look at the point, and visualize your goals.

After you complete eagle pose on the other side, fly your body out of the pose by releasing your leg outward and both of your arms out and up. Circle your arms overhead and bring your hands together, with your thumbs at the third eye. Spread apart the skin of the forehead here to complete the Wayne Cook posture. Then press your fingertips into the center of your forehead and spread apart the skin. Release your hands to your side, pause, and relax.

Inversions

In the science of yoga-pose sequencing (vinyasa krama), standing poses are followed by inversions. If you practice headstand or shoulderstand or handstand, you'll insert them into your practice template after standing poses. You do them at this point so there is enough time in your practice to counter the cervical vertebral stress, as well as to calm the nervous system down after the excitement and energy intensity of inversions.

The inversions we do in Energy Medicine Yoga could more properly be considered restoratives. Therefore, they come later in the practice, before the relaxation poses. In some traditions, like Ashtanga, the intense inversions are practiced at the end of the class to increase lucidity in savasana.

Backbends

Camel Pose (*Ustrasana*) with Meridian Point Holds

Camel pose is a great backbend that is good for beginners as well as the most advanced practitioner. Because you are on your knees, it helps to stabilize the hips and is a good way to learn how to keep the vertebrae of the low back from compressing.

Start on your knees with your toes tucked under. Bring your hands into triple warmer/heart mudra in front of the chest. Lift the chest up and press the chest into the hands as you start to lean back. Keep pressing the hips forward as well, trying to keep the hips directly over the knees. Think about lengthening up the spine as you're leaning back. Continue looking forward for this first preparation part of the pose. Take three to five deep breaths, and then slowly lift the body up and release back down onto the haunches.

If that much was challenging, continue to work with the preparation part of the pose until the spine is strengthened and toned. If that much was easeful for you, consider deepening the pose. The next time you lift up and open the spine, bend back as if you're bending over a beach ball. Reach the hands down to the feet. Take your thumbs and press them deeply into the hollows on the insides of the Achilles tendons. This helps activate the arms and the upper body, making the bend in the upper back lighter and more open.

Your thumbs are pressing into the kidney 3 (K-3) points, which are the source points for the kidney meridian. They are considered the source points of all source points. Source points connect the meridian energy directly to the organ they feed, nourishing and energizing that organ. In the case of K-3, not only are you sending powerful energy to the kidneys, but you're also helping meridian energy feed all of the organs. Because this pose is a backbend, you are also gently squeezing and releasing the kidneys themselves, helping to flush and cleanse them. Holding K-3 in this pose is a powerful aid to help cleanse the hardest-working cleansing organs in your body.

When you're ready to release, slowly lift up out of the backbend and come to sit back on your heels. Take a few breaths in preparation for the next lift.

The next time you lift up, move your thumbs to the outsides of the Achilles tendons, and your fingers will come around to the inside of your heels. This hand position creates an outward rotation of your upper arms, opening up the whole upper back.

Opposite K-3 on the outside of the Achilles tendon is the point bladder 60. The bladder meridian rules the nervous system, is connected to all the organs, and brings energy to fuel the brain. (It is the longest meridian, going from the top of the head, down the back and legs, and off the toes.) The bladder 60 point in particular helps activate the back body, which is important in a backbend. Many times in backbends, we actually collapse the back instead of energize it. Holding this point, as we're doing here, helps to counter that collapse by sending energy up the spine.

Hold for five to seven breaths and release.

You can do this pose again, releasing the tops of the feet to the floor to access an even deeper bend. Continue to move the hips forward. If you feel very comfortable with this pose, you can begin the pose with your hands on K-3 and then press the hips up. Just remember to open up the lower back by lifting the spine up and over an imaginary ball at your back. There should be no compression in the low spine. You can also release your head back if your neck feels comfortable.

When you're complete, release down onto your heels and cup the back of one palm into the other on your lap. Relax here in this mudra of completion for several breaths.

Pigeon Pose (*Eka Pada Rajakapotanasana*) with Neurovascular Hold

This is a wonderful backbend into a deep relaxation. Starting either in downward dog or on all fours, bring your right knee forward and place it in between your hands. The outside of the knee and leg will be on the floor. The knee can be deeply bent, or, if you're more flexible, going toward a 90-degree angle, with the right foot and right knee spanning between the hands. This position calls for a deep outward rotation in the thigh.

Press down firmly on the ground with the hands and lift up through the heart center. Try to keep your hips equally balanced. You may want to slide some padding, such as a folded blanket, under your right hip to keep yourself from leaning over to the right side. You can tuck the toes of the left foot under to extend that heel back and to help stabilize the pose. Stay here and breathe until you feel the hips relax and open.

After you've opened up the shoulders and back, lean forward and continue to open up the hips while resting the upper body on a bolster, a block, or your hands. You can uncurl the toes of your left foot.

No matter what your head is resting on, bring your forehead into your open palms. You can either use one palm across the whole forehead or put both palms on your forehead with the fingertips reaching into the hairline. You are stimulating the main neurovascular points, which Donna calls the "Oh my God" points. These points, located on the frontal protuberance of the forehead, help to keep blood in the forebrain. During any stressful experience (including

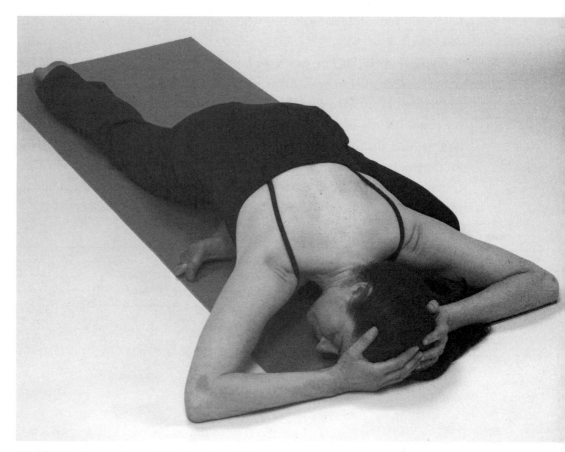

FIGURE 44   **Pigeon Pose with Rooster Comb Hold**

stress-inducing yoga poses), the blood tends to leave the forebrain in preparation for fight-or-flight. The blood goes to the extremities and stops being available for normal cognitive processes. By holding the hands over these points, you keep the blood in the brain and available for creative and intelligent thinking. You'll learn more about these points in the appendix. Any time that you're resting your head in any yoga pose, hold your forehead in this way. (Conversely, resting your forehead on the backs of your hands helps to balance your polarity with the polarity of the earth, a very simple way to bring yourself into concert with the earth's energies.)

VARIATION: PIGEON WITH ROOSTER COMB HOLD

Another option in pigeon pose is the rooster comb hold, which helps to stimulate and balance the hypothalamus, pituitary, and pineal glands. We'll also use this hold in our savasana preparation, and you can experiment with doing this hold when you're folded forward or when you're lying on your back to see which you prefer.

In pigeon pose, slightly turn your head toward the front foot. Bring the heel of one hand to the forehead. Allow the fingers to come up and over the head to rest on the crown. Take your other hand and bring the heel of it to the back of your head, directly behind your brows. Allow the fingers to come up and over the head to meet the fingers of the other hand on the crown. (See figure 44.) Hold for three minutes. This hold stimulates all the master glands and brings them into communication with each other. There is also the added benefit of holding the liver neurovascular points, because liver metabolizes all the hormones.

Twists and Seated Poses

Seated Forward Bend (*Paschimottanasana*) with Neurolymphatic Cleanse and Gallbladder Neurovascular Hold

Sometimes working the neurolymphatic reflex points while standing is more challenging than working them in seated or supine poses. This pose is an alternative way to clear the neurolymphatic reflex points on the legs, helping you to increase your forward fold and to detoxify.

Sit on the floor with both legs extended in front of you. Reach underneath your butt and move the flesh out of the way, so the sitting bones are more directly on the floor. If you have a pronounced backward curve in the low back, due to tight hips, elevate the hips by sitting on some folded blankets.

Inhale, and extend the arms overhead. Exhale, and fold over the legs, weaving your hands in a figure eight as you fold. Make sure the fold is coming from the hips and not the upper back or the waist. Inhale and sit up again; exhale and fold forward. Do this two more times. Inhale back up to sitting.

Now bring your fingers and thumbs of both hands into the three-point notch, and vigorously massage the pinstripe lines on the outsides of your thighs—the large-intestine neurolymphatic points. And then massage on the inside seam of the thighs—the small-intestine neurolymphatic points and circulation-sex neurolymphatic points. You can massage one leg at a time, working up or down the thigh with one hand on each seam. Remember to work from the knee up if you tend toward loose stools, and work from the hips down if you tend toward constipation. (See figure 6 in part 1.)

When you're finished, inhale the arms up overhead, and exhale, folding over the legs. Hold for one to three minutes. If you can easily reach your feet in this position, you can pulse or hold onto the kidney 1 point in the center of the ball of the foot. This is deeply grounding and nourishing.

If you can't reach the feet, slide your hands underneath the back of the knees. Hold here gently as you fold forward. Behind the knees are three gallbladder neurovascular reflex points, three of the few neurovasculars that aren't on the head. Gallbladder neurovasculars are emotional balancers. The gallbladder meridian's peak or high-tide time of day comes just after that of triple warmer. Holding the gallbladder neurovascular points takes the yang energy out of triple warmer and helps to calm it. Notice how you feel after holding these points.

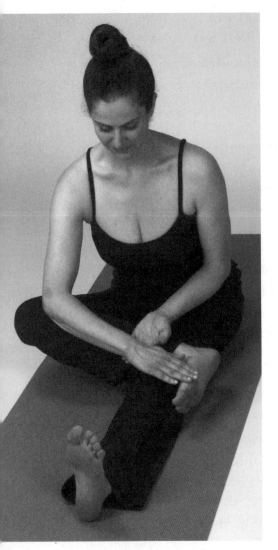

FIGURE 45   Half Ankle-to-Knee Pose (Ardha Agnistambhasana) with Circulation-Sex Sedation

Half Ankle-to-Knee Pose (Ardha Agnistambhasana) with Circulation-Sex Sedation

The circulation-sex meridian governs the hips and the reproductive organs, as well as the protective layer of the heart, called the pericardium. This meridian taps directly into the root chakra and connects to all the other chakras, calming and relaxing them. It also helps to relax the hips on a physical level and to dissipate the emotional component of tight hips, which is often related to a sexual imbalance. Sedating the circulation-sex meridian also has a systemic, balancing effect on all the other meridians that help to balance the hormones. Indeed, the spleen, kidney, and circulation-sex meridians are three of the eight meridians that most affect the hormones.

Donna has said that most people need to sedate the circulation-sex meridian; however, if you feel off after doing the sedating, you may need to follow it with strengthening. I've included both sets of points, sedating and strengthening, in the circulation-sex exercise if you want to use them. If you do both sedating and strengthening, you should also use the control points afterward. We'll start with circulation-sex sedating, because doing this affects all the other meridians. And by helping to open and relax the hips, it makes forward folds and hip openers easier.

Sit on the floor, and extend your left leg. Bend your right leg and cross the right ankle over the left thigh, just above the knee. You can lift the hips off the floor slightly by sitting on a folded blanket.

Take your right hand and cover spleen 3 on the right foot. (For the exact location of spleen 3, see the instructions for the Kidney Three-Point Pose in week 4. This point is also a control point for the kidney meridian.) Take your left hand and cover circulation-sex 7, located in the center of the right inner-wrist crease.

As you hold these two points, lean forward over your legs, bending at the hips, not the back. (See figure 45.) You may start to feel pulsing under your fingers at the points. Eventually, the pulsing will synchronize and strengthen. This is the meridian energy synching up and doing its job. Don't worry if you don't feel it; after about three minutes, the energy will be connected even if you don't feel it. Eventually, after you practice for some time, you'll start to feel this energy. You won't be uncertain when you feel it for the first time. It is powerful!

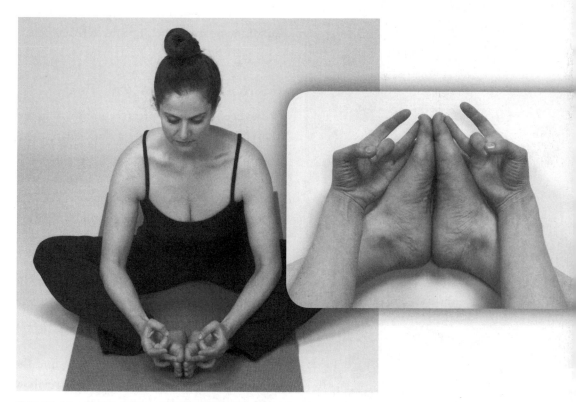

FIGURE 46   Cobbler's Pose with Circulation-Sex Strengthening

After three minutes, switch sides.

If you've decided to do circulation-sex meridian strengthening as well, you'll do that now. Come into cobbler's pose, with the soles of the feet together and knees out to the side. Put the fourth finger onto liver 1, on the inside edge of the big-toe toenail. Take your thumbs and hold the tip of the middle finger on the edge closest to the thumb. (See figure 46.) You can hold the points on both feet and hands at the same time. Again, hold these points for three minutes.

To hold the circulation-sex control points, your right leg will be extended, and your left leg bent at the knee with the ankle over the right thigh. Hold kidney 10, at the edge of the fold in the left knee, with your left hand. Hold circulation-sex 3, at the center of the inside elbow crease, with your right hand. (See figure 47.) Maintain the hold for about a minute and a half and then switch sides.

See figure 48 for the locations of all the circulation-sex strengthening and sedating points.

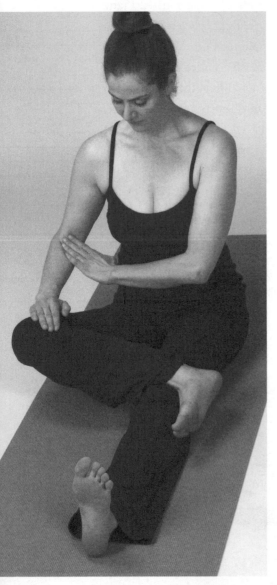

FIGURE 47   Half Ankle-to-Knee Pose with Circulation-Sex Control Points

Source-Point Mudra Walk: Feet

We've been using acupressure points to access the meridians to strengthen and sedate them. But there are also points along the meridians called *source points,* which are used to send energy directly to the organ associated with that meridian (as we learned with K-3). I use source points in several ways. Some of you may be familiar with "the headache point." This point, large intestine 4, is located against the bone of the index finger, where the finger and thumb joint meet. If you apply deep pressure here, you can alleviate a headache.

In the meditation section, you can find the source-point mudra walk for the hands. Following is the source-point mudra walk for the feet.

Note: the points large intestine 4 (the headache point) and kidney 3 are not to be used during pregnancy, as both have the potential to induce labor.

Half hero (*ardha virasana*) with kidney and bladder source points. Start in half hero pose, with your left leg extended and your right knee bent back, with the right foot coming to rest next to the right hip. This can be an intense stretch, and you can sit on the edge of a blanket to take the intensity out of the knee.

We start the mudra walk with the water-element meridians. When doing healing work on the meridians, you always start in water, the kidney being the birthplace of the meridians and the place from which they all emerge. The kidney source point is the master source point; it sends energy anywhere it is needed. (Note: using this point is contraindicated for pregnant women.)

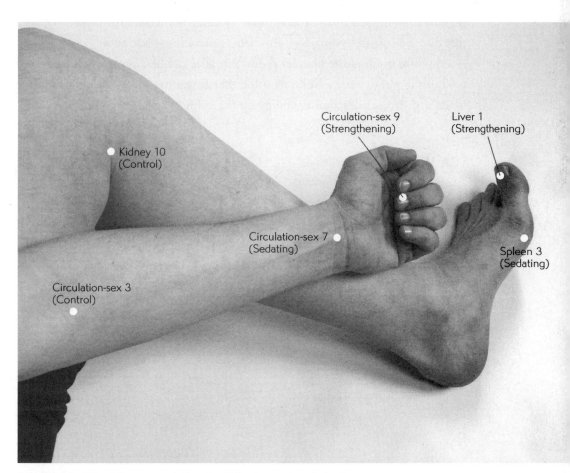

FIGURE 48   Circulation-sex sedating, strengthening, and control points

The first source points on the mudra walk are kidney 3 (K-3) and bladder 64. K-3 is located directly behind the anklebone, in the hollow of the Achilles tendon on the big-toe side of the foot. (See figure 16.) Bladder 64 is located directly in front of (toward the toes) the protruding bone halfway down the outside edge of your foot. (See figures 49 and 50.) You can tap these points, massage them deeply, or simply hold them and wait for the pulses to come up and synchronize. Hold K-3 with your thumb and wrap the hand around to hold bladder 64 with your pinky or ring finger. By working both these points together, you are energizing and strengthening both the yin and the yang of the water element, bringing them into balance.

As you're holding the points, visualize your kidneys. See the actual organs, located on either side of the small of your back, at the height of the waist. The right kidney is slightly lower then the left one. They are a bit larger than the size of your fist. Their main physiological job is to filter waste from the blood and to manufacture urine. As you're holding the kidney points, see the organ receiving this direct energy. Holding K-3 also helps relieve low-back pain.

As you're holding the bladder point, visualize the bladder itself. It is located behind the pubic bone and holds urine that is waiting to be released. Holding bladder points sends calming energy up the spine.

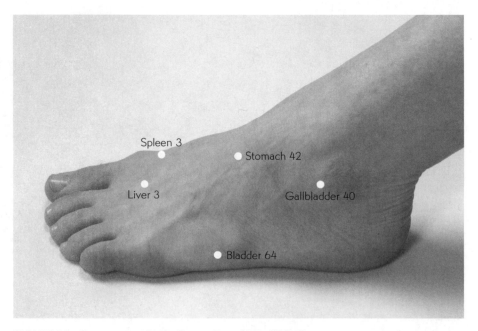

FIGURE 49   **Source points for the Source-Point Mudra Walk: Feet**

When you're complete on the first side, straighten the right leg, bend the left leg back, and hold kidney 3 and bladder 64 on the left foot.

Tip: If you're comfortable in full hero's pose, you can hold both sets of points on both feet at the same time.

From water we move to wood.

Forward-bending twist (*marichiasana* I) with liver and gallbladder source points. Bring the left foot back down to the floor with the knee up in the air. The right leg will remain extended. The meridians for wood are liver and gallbladder. Liver 3 is located an inch back from the gully where the big toe and first toe meet, between the metatarsal bones. Gallbladder 40 is located in front of the anklebone on the outside of the foot in the dip toward the bottom of the foot. (If the anklebone is a quadrant, the dip is in the lower-left square.)

Again, hold, massage, tap, or pulse these points. (See figure 51.) Your right hand will reach out and hold the big toe of your right foot in yogic toe lock.

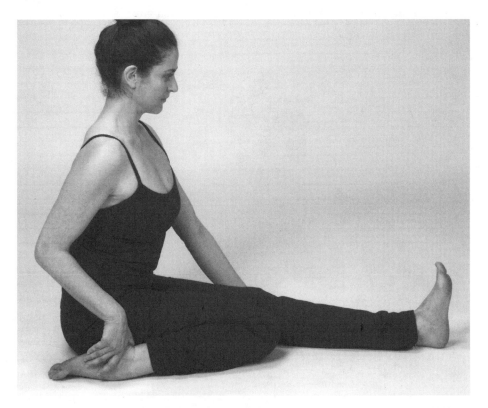

FIGURE 50   Source-Point Mudra Walk: Feet, half hero (ardha virasana) with kidney and bladder source points

(See week 4 for details about why the yogic toe lock is important.) If you can't reach your right foot, bring your hand behind the knee and hold the gallbladder neurovascular points. This pose resembles an archer holding back the bow.

As you're holding, visualize your liver. This is the yin, wood organ, working all the time, as the yin organs do. It is attached to the bottom of the diaphragm and almost completely fills the upper-right abdominal region and the top of the left region. The liver stores and regulates blood volume; breaks down toxic substances, including alcohol; and creates and stores amino acids, proteins, and fats and cholesterol, which are used in the creation of hormones. These are just some of its functions. The liver is the only organ that has the ability to regenerate itself, so it is appropriate that it is the organ of spring, which is all about rebirth and new life.

The gallbladder is a pear-shaped organ connected to the underside of the liver. It stores extra bile to be released to aid in the digestion of fats.

When you are complete on the first side, transition to the other side, maintaining contact with either the liver and gallbladder points or the yogic toe lock as you do so. You can straighten the left leg and switch your fingers to yogic toe

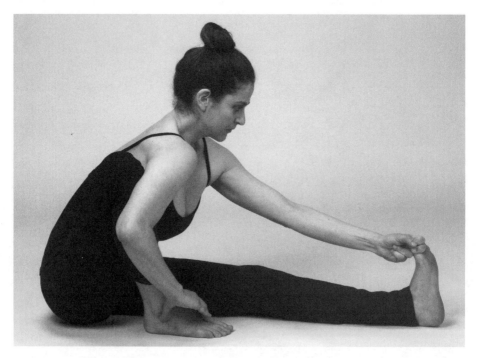

FIGURE 51   Source-Point Mudra Walk: Feet, forward-bending twist (marichiasana I) with liver and gallbladder source points

lock; then pull your right leg in by pulling back on the big toe, and switch to hold liver 3 and gallbladder 40 when the foot is in place. Hold the second side as long as you held the first.

Seated forward bend (paschimottanasana) with stomach and spleen source points. When you've completed the wood meridians, you'll move to the earth element and the stomach and spleen meridians. If you can't reach your toes in full forward bend, bring your feet to your body in cobbler's pose. In either position, wrap your hands around your feet, with your thumb draping just below the ball of the foot; this is spleen 3. Your hand should span over the highest point of the top of the foot; that point is stomach 42. (See figure 52.) You can hold both these points on both feet at the same time, lending a cohesion and a closing to this moving mudra.

While you're holding these points, visualize the spleen, the yin, earth organ. The spleen is located on the left side of the body, high up in the abdomen.

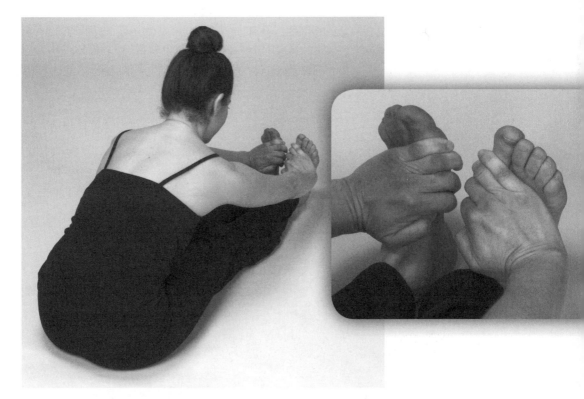

FIGURE 52   Source-Point Mudra Walk: Feet, seated forward bend (paschimottanasana) with stomach and spleen source points

The spleen filters and cleans the blood, as well as clearing bacteria and toxins from the body. It also produces lymph cells and stores blood for additional body demands. The stomach takes up the rest of the space in the left upper body cavity. Nestled under the diaphragm and between the left lobe of the liver and the spleen, it holds food during its breakdown stage and then moves food through the digestive tract.

When you're complete with this hold, shake out your legs and shake off your hands briskly.

Reclining Poses, Restorative Inversions, and Relaxation Preparation

Laughing Baby Pose (*Ananda Balasana*) with K-1 Massage

Lie on your back and pull your knees in toward your armpits, with your legs bent at 90-degree angles, so the feet look like they could walk on the ceiling. Even though you're pulling your legs in, try to extend through the spine, pressing your low back to the floor. This oppositional stretch helps open the hips even more. Reach your hands to your feet and gently pull the knees deeper into the armpits. Alternately, if it feels more comfortable, you can pull the knees outside the armpits toward the floor.

Squeeze around the widest part of the foot. This helps to stimulate and awaken radiant circuit energy. Next deeply press in and massage K-1, the first point of kidney meridian. Now pulse it, pressing and releasing, pressing and releasing. The point is located where the ball of the big toe meets the ball of the second/third toes, in that slight indentation. This is the entry point of earth energy into the body. It is called the "Wellspring of Life" point, and pulsing it resets the energy systems of the whole body.

Upward-Facing Triple Diamond Pose with Electrics

Another lovely way to use the electrics is in upward-facing triple diamond pose. This pose is a deep hip and heart opener. The teacher who taught me this pose said it is for releasing anger and greed. You can simply bring to mind anything that resonates with you in those realms, and let it release as your body is responding to this electrical influx.

Lie on your back, with the soles of your feet together, knees out to the sides. This is the first diamond. Bring your arms overhead, elbows out to the side. This is the second diamond. Now bring your thumbs into the electric points at the back of the head (see week 6), and interlace your fingers under your head as a cushion. Your hands, connected to your head, form the third diamond. (See figure 53.) Allow yourself to surrender and release into the pose as you breathe deeply into the belly.

When you feel complete, slowly straighten the bends in the body, stretching long as you do so.

Downward-Facing Triple Diamond Pose with Third-Eye Hold

This downward-facing form of the triple diamond pose is to release sadness and grief. Allow any emotions to leave you, entering the floor and the earth, where everything can be grounded.

Lie on your stomach. Bring the soles of the feet together, knees out to the sides; this is the first diamond. Bring your hands above your head with the thumbs and index fingers together; this is the second diamond. The third diamond is formed by your bent elbows.

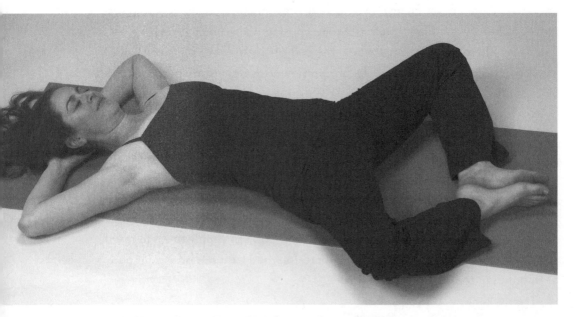

FIGURE 53   Upward-Facing Triple Diamond Pose with Electrics

Rest the forehead on the thumbs, with the tips of the thumbs in the indent at the top of the nose, where it meets the forehead at the area of the third eye. Adjust until you find a comfortable place for the head. Release the jaw completely, letting the lower teeth fall forward. (See figure 54.)

This is a deep hip opener, and lots of emotion can arise from it. Just breathe into the belly, letting it lift the body off the floor, and let yourself release as much as possible.

When you feel complete with this pose, slowly straighten the bends of the body, stretching along the floor. Rock the sacrum back and forth to calm triple warmer and further release tension and stress.

Plow Pose (*Halasana*) with Gallbladder Neurovasculars and Calf Massage

Another gentle yet powerful inversion is the plow pose (halasana). This pose is often practiced with the same setup for shoulderstand: a folded blanket under the shoulders, with the head off the blanket to allow room for the neck to extend and not compress. But there are many variations of this pose, and you can still receive the benefits even with most of your back on the floor and only

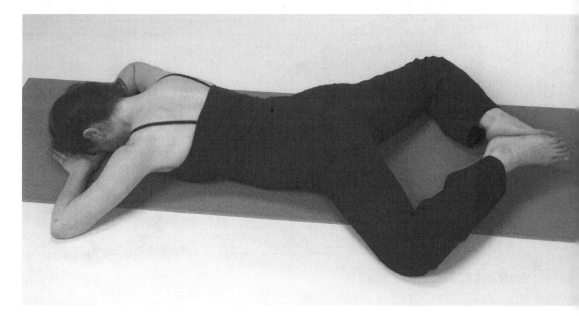

FIGURE 54   Downward-Facing Triple Diamond Pose with Third-Eye Hold

your legs folded over you. This is like seated forward bend (paschimottanasana), but upside down. In the Energy Medicine Yoga version of plow, you will work some very powerful points on the lower legs. Lie on your back, with or without padding under the shoulders (but not under the head). Use your hands pressed on the floor, as well as your stomach muscles, to lift your legs up and fold them back over your body. If you're more flexible, you can bring the legs all the way overhead until the toes reach the ground. You can also just bring the legs over the body.

Now reach to the largest, fleshiest part of the calf and start to massage it, focusing on the lowest, diminishing part of the muscle. This muscle is called the soleus. It is considered to be the second heart because it is responsible for sending venous blood back to the heart and the brain. This muscle is often sore and tight, and massaging it is crucial for keeping it supple and working well. This inversion, which is already helping ease the flow of venous blood, is a great time to work this muscle.

After you finish massaging the soleus, work your way down to the ankle and massage there. You'll end up on the Achilles tendon. The ankle and Achilles

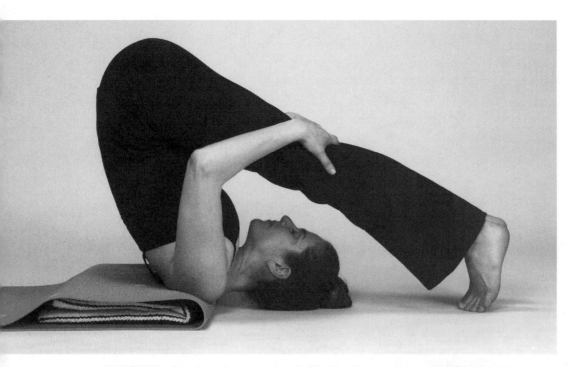

FIGURE 55   Plow Pose (halasana) with Gallbladder Neurovasculars and Calf Massage

are part of the tendon guard reflex, which is a reflex deeply related to the fight-or-flight response and to communication. A shortened Achilles tendon has been linked to learning disabilities and to difficulty communicating. Studies have shown that lengthening this tendon can help with communication. High-heeled shoes can also shorten this tendon, and so if you wear high heels regularly, make sure to work the calves even more. After massaging here, hold and squeeze the Achilles tendon. This stimulates both the K-3 and bladder 60 points. (See the instructions for Camel Pose [Ustrasana] with Meridian Point Holds in the backbends chapter for more on these important points.)

Now bring both hands to the backs of the knees and hold there. These are the gallbladder neurovascular points (figure 55). These points are intimately connected to triple warmer, as the gallbladder meridian both feeds triple warmer energy and is fed energy by triple warmer. Gallbladder rules decisions, and when it is out of balance, it can be characterized by anger and rash decision-making or indecision and timidity. Balancing this meridian can help make decision-making easier. The gallbladder meridian distributes energy through the body, and when you're balancing the neurovascular points of gallbladder, the heart meridian energy also balances. As explained in week 4 of part 1, each meridian has a two-hour cycle during which it is at the height of its energy. When the energy of gallbladder is at its height, the energy of heart is at its weakest. So by balancing and energizing gallbladder's energy, you help keep it from stealing heart energy, thereby allowing heart to balance also.

The gallbladder neurovasculars are also emotional balancers, as noted in the directions for Seated Forward Bend (Paschimottanasana) with Neurolymphatic Cleanse and Gallbladder Neurovascular Hold in the chapter on twists and seated poses. Gallbladder is at its peak energy in the two hours just after triple warmer's two-hour peak, and holding gallbladder's neurovasculars takes the yang, intense energy out of triple warmer, helping to calm it. Gallbladder is also the digester of what seems impossible, bringing you the strength to do challenging work. Holding these points is deeply soothing and energizing to the whole body, both physically and emotionally.

When you feel complete, slowly roll down from the pose, bending your knees to release the feet to the floor. Lift and lower the hips a few times in conjunction with your breath, to release the lower back. You can also fold the knees into the chest and hug them tight to finish this practice.

Tip: This entire calf sequence can also easily be done in laughing baby pose.

Closing Your Physical Practice:
Eye Yoga and Savasana

Eye Yoga

I remember doing eye yoga when I was in my teacher training and hating it. I thought it was so slow and boring. But as I learned more and more about the eyes and their connection to healing, I became a devotee of some of these more esoteric practices.

"The eyes are the windows to the soul"—a truer statement could not be made. On a very gross level, the eyes contain a blueprint for what is going on in all the other tissues of the body. Learning to read this blueprint is the study of iridology. Just as the foot and hand both contain reflex points for the rest of the body, so, too, do the eyes. The visual system (which includes your eyes and their supporting nerves and tissues) uses more than 25 percent of the nutrients that you absorb from food. The eyes also hold 80 percent of the tension of the body, so relaxing the eyes has an enormous overall effect.

The following eye-yoga exercises help tone the optic nerve and, by working the eye muscles, increase circulation to the delicate tissues and nerves that make up the eye itself. Doing these can help improve eyesight and release stress and trauma. You can do these exercises when you lie down on your back, immediately before savasana.

COMPASS GAZING (*NETHRA VYAYAMAM*) AND PALMING

You can do these exercises in a comfortable seated position or lying on your back on the floor. Make sure you are moving only your eyes and not your head. Move slowly and deliberately. Don't rush.

First, open your eyes and look up as far as you can. Come back to center and look down as far as you can. Come back to center and look as far as you can to the left. Come back to center and look as far as you can to the right. Come back to center.

Now look diagonally, first up to the right and then down to the left. Come back to center. Look diagonally up to the left and then down to the right. Come back to center.

Now slowly work your eyes around in a circle clockwise. (Although the pose is named after a compass, it might make more sense to name it for a clock. It involves a similar idea of following details around in a circle.) Start by looking up at a twelve o'clock position, then move your eyes around to three o'clock, down to six o'clock, around to nine o'clock, and back to twelve. Do this two more times. Keep your breath slow and steady. Notice if there are any areas of tension or constriction. If one area is difficult, spend a bit of time going back and forth over it.

Then circle the eyes several times in the counterclockwise direction. Again, if there is tension or difficulty or the breath becomes ragged, try to relax and remain on the challenging point. You can bring one hand to the frontal neurovascular points on the forehead to help dissolve any stress you may feel when you find a place of tension.

After you've finished circles, take one hand and, with your fingers in a three-point notch an inch or two in front of your face, trace a figure-eight pattern in front of your eyes, crossing in between the eyes. As you draw the figure eight, follow your fingers with your eyes. Go slowly. Again, if this action feels stressful or challenging, bring your other hand to the forehead to cover the neurovascular points there.

After you've finished, rub your hands together, generating heat, and cup them over your closed eyes. The heel of the hand is on the cheekbone, and the palm is over the eye cavity, but not touching the eye. Hold here for several breaths. You can actually hold this position for quite a long time, and the longer you hold it, the deeper the relaxation response and benefit to the eyes. This technique, called palming, is used quite extensively in natural vision-healing programs. The heat and electromagnetism from your hands help to relax the muscles that move the eye and to energize the delicate eyeball tissue.

Natural vision therapy pioneer Meir Schneider healed his eyes completely from severe cataracts and botched surgeries that left him legally blind. At the outset, he would palm them for several hours a day.

OTHER EYE YOGA TECHNIQUES

Tapping and pinching the orbital bone. First lightly tap and then pinch, with a very soft and small touch, around the orbital bone surrounding the eye. Then do the same with the eyelid. This releases stuck energies and rebalances the vision in both eyes.

Tapping the eyeball. Lay one finger over the closed eyelid and gently tap on it with the other hand. This helps with eye fatigue and creates a wave that pulses all the way to the back side of the head and upward throughout the brain, connecting energy patterns to the optic nerve and releasing eye strain.

Clearing meridian points around the eyes. Liver, kidney, and stomach are the three primary meridians associated with the eyes. Clearing the lymph, as we did in Triangle Pose (Trikonasana) with SLK and Stomach Line Clear (standing poses chapter) and in the Kidney Three-Point Pose (week 4), is wonderful for the eyes. The fourth of the Four Thumps (week 1), which taps the stomach-meridian point beneath the eye, and the Crown Pull (week 1) are also good techniques for helping the eyes.

If eye yoga is something you want to work with more, there are many wonderful natural vision-therapy resources available. There are also many traditions that believe the eyes hold our patterns and contain our trauma. Techniques such as EMDR work with this concept and can be very powerful. Tracing the figure-eight pattern while holding the forehead neurovascular points, as we did above, is similar to some of the EMDR work for releasing trauma, but much more basic.

Deep Relaxation: Savasana with Rooster Comb Hold

Savasana is considered the most difficult pose in yoga. Many students skip it completely, sneaking out of class before savasana or not including it in their home practice. Savasana is the time, however, when the real benefits of the yoga practice take hold. In this pose, when the body is deeply relaxed, the cells absorb the work.

This is also the pose where we experience and practice dying—hence the name *corpse pose*. We essentially die to this moment, letting the moment pass by without grasping it, and allow the new moment to arise. It's a time where we can experiment with the transience of the physical body, knowing that we are not the body. So what are we? It is in this time out of time that those ideas can germinate, returning you to yourself new and less attached to the false idea of permanence.

As you're getting ready to end the practice with savasana, you come to a quieter mind.

The Rooster Comb Hold, which is also used in the backbends chapter with pigeon pose (eka pada rajakapotanasana), is something you'll do again here in preparation for savasana. After you try it in both poses, you'll find if you prefer to do this hold while folded forward (in pigeon) or while lying on your back (in savasana). Again, the rooster comb hold balances all your hormones. It balances the interplay between the hypothalamus, which is considered to be the master gland, and the pineal and the pituitary glands. The neurovascular points for the liver meridian, the big metabolizer for the hormones, are also held.

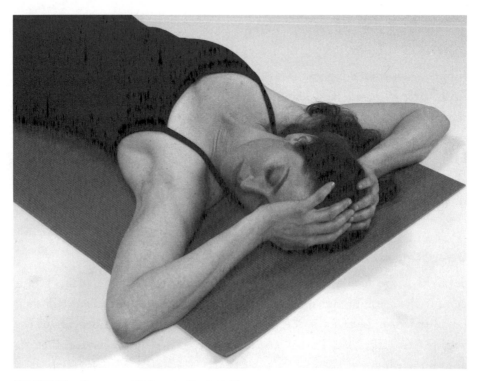

FIGURE 56   Savasana with Rooster Comb Hold

Lie down on your back in savasana. Turn your head slightly to one side and bring the heel of one hand to the forehead. Drape the fingers over the top of the head. Take your other hand and either put the heel of that hand on the top of the head, where the fingertips of the other hand end, or place the fingertips of the second hand next to the fingertips of the first and drape the heel over the upper back of the head. Either way, you'll be covering the points on the front and back of the head. (See figure 56.)

Hold these points for anywhere from one to ten minutes. When you feel complete, release your hands to the sides, and continue to rest in savasana.

Meditation

Meditation is a simple tool that can change your life in dramatic ways. There are so many reasons to meditate, and more and more studies are coming out about the value and power of meditation. People use it to reduce stress, lower blood pressure, and increase concentration and performance in a variety of disciplines. It seems odd that sitting still and focusing the mind on one thing, like the breath or a mantra, could help you in every other area of your life. But the studies are powerful.

If you want to understand how your mind works so you can begin to dismantle behaviors that aren't serving you, meditation is the tool for you. If you want to bring more calm and contentment to your life, connect more to your intuition and with the world, and experience your own divinity, meditation is your practice. Do a bit of your own research to discover the many benefits of this practice, and I encourage you to bring it into your life.

You can practice meditation after savasana or on its own, first thing when you get up in the morning, at noon, or last thing before you go to bed. Those are the ideal times to practice. The most auspicious time is between 3:30 and 5:00 in the morning, before the day begins, just as dawn is breaking. This is also the high tide of lung meridian, where you have the most access to the breath. My teacher says this is the best time to practice meditation. The next best time to practice is whenever you can!

Simply sitting still and watching the breath, or focusing on a Sanskrit mantra such as *Ham Sa* or *So Hum,* can be a very easy and accessible way to begin.

A general rule of thumb is that twenty minutes a day is necessary to maintain a balanced and equanimous life. But to begin, five minutes is a good place to start. At the end of a week, add another five minutes, until eventually you are up to twenty. If you have more time and want to take your practice deeper, you can build up to forty-five minutes or an hour.

Breath Meditation

The most basic and widespread meditation technique is simply to watch your breath. Although I say, "simply," once you try watching your breath, you will see how challenging it can be. And that challenge is part of the process. By slowing down your breath, body, and mind, you begin to see how your mind works and begin to create space around your egoic preferences and drives. You become calmer, more centered, better able to make informed decisions, more in touch with your intuition, and eventually able to feel your connection to the oneness of the universe.

Begin by sitting in a comfortable position. You can sit on the floor with some cushions underneath your sitting bones to lift the hips above the knees. You can sit on a chair with your feet planted flat on the floor. You can also do meditation lying down, if sitting presents a challenge.

Close the eyes and begin to watch your breath. You can focus on the nostrils, feeling the air as it moves into the body. You can watch the rise and fall of the chest or the expansion and contraction of the abdomen. You can listen to the sound of your breath in your ears or feel the breath with your inner senses. If your mind starts to wander, gently bring it back to your breath. If thoughts arise, think of them like clouds passing by in the sky, without fixating on any of them. Trust that if a thought is important, it will come back when you are ready to deal with it. The most powerful studies I've seen show that the importance of meditation practice comes from seeing that the mind is wandering and bringing it back to the breath. That moment is the one that trains the mind. And this mind training is actually training you to be happier, more content, and more empowered in your life.

Mantra Meditation

Sometimes, the mind is so busy that it seems impossible to quiet it, even for a moment. This is called the monkey mind, as it seems to be jumping from thought to thought to thought, like a monkey soaring from branch to branch and tree to tree. If this is the case, the breath may not be a strong enough focal point to keep you grounded. You can use a simple mantra to begin to discipline the mind.

A mantra is a word or phrase that you repeat in the silence of your mind. The most often prescribed mantra for a beginning meditator is the phrase *So Hum* or *Ham Sa*. Each is basically the same phrase in reverse, one that means "I am that" or "It is so." It has no religious or deity-based significance. It is simply a declaration that you are here, in this body, sitting still. The Sanskrit language is a resonance language, which means the vibration of the words actually affects you at a cellular level. It doesn't matter if you know what the words mean; your body responds regardless. This is one of the reasons chanting is so popular and powerful in the yogic tradition. It transforms you. So saying this mantra has a powerful effect on your body, as well as giving the mind something to do.

If you want to work with more mantras, I suggest the book *The Power of Mantra and the Mystery of Initiation,* by Pandit Rajmani Tigunait (see the bibliography). There are many mantras available on the Internet, but not all of them will be appropriate to use. Find a good and qualified teacher to help take you deeper into mantra-meditation practice.

Source-Point Mudra Walk: Hands

I love this meditation, as it helps to focus the mind, giving it a point of contact. Using the source-point mudra is sort of like using *mala* beads, which are beads used to help practice mantra meditation. Here, the mudra serves as the point of focus.

One of the most common, widely used, and powerful mudras is chin mudra. It is the mudra most often used for meditation practice. It is the linking of the index finger with the thumb. The index finger represents individual will, and the thumb, universal will. With this mudra, you bow the individual will to the universal will.

I also love the energetic component of the mudra, which is rarely taught. The tip of the thumb is the end of the lung meridian, the yin metal element, and the tip of the index finger is the start of the large-intestine meridian, the yang metal element. Connecting these two meridians actually runs the energy cycle of these two metal elements, the element of letting go. Lung runs over the lungs and off the thumb, and large intestine runs up the arm, starting at the index finger and ending below the nostril. It is the perfect connection to help amplify the ease of breath and allow the body to let go both emotionally and energetically.

The Source-Point Mudra Walk on the hands follows a similar path for connecting the elements. The meridians in the hands relate to metal, as we've seen with lung and large intestine, and also fire. Fire relates to both inspiration and anxiety. By holding these points in meditation, you are both calming anxiety and balancing inspiration. You are also working directly with the organs by using the source points. With this mudra, you activate the physical small intestine, heart and pericardium, lungs, and large intestine. Triple warmer is the only meridian involved in the mudra that does not have a corresponding organ.

You'll begin with the triple warmer–circulation-sex connection. Sit in your comfortable meditative seat, either in a chair or on a meditation cushion. With your left hand resting palm up, bring the middle finger of your right hand to triple warmer 4, and the thumb to circulation-sex 7. Triple warmer 4 is located on the back of the wrist, in the slight dip at the wrist crease, in between the large tendon of the pinky finger and the joined group of tendons from the first, second, and third fingers. Circulation-sex 7 is located at the center of the front wrist crease, in line with the middle finger (figure 57).

Hold the two points until the pulses beat together. (This pulse can be the focus of your meditation.) At the same time, visualize the pericardium, which is the muscle that protects the heart and keeps the heart rhythm in synch. Triple warmer controls all three regions of the abdomen, so you could also focus on the balanced heat distribution through your core. After you feel the pulses of the points beating together and strongly, move to the next set of points.

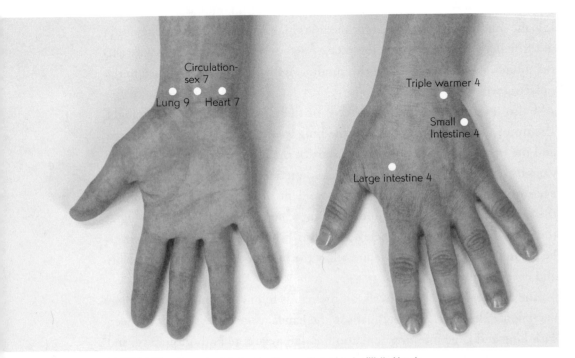

FIGURE 57   Source points for the Source-Point Mudra Walk: Hands

Hold small intestine 4 with the middle finger and heart 7 with the thumb. To find small intestine 4, slide your middle finger down the long bone at the side of the hand (the karate-chop bone); just as this bone meets the top of the wrist joint, there is a small dip. This is small intestine 4. Heart 7 is located at the front crease of the wrist, just inside the last tendon, in line with the pinky (figure 57).

Again, hold these points. Visualize the heart. Maybe you can feel it beating in your body. See the oxygenated blood come in and the de-oxygenated blood go out. See the small intestine. It starts its attachment at the stomach and fills most of the abdominal cavity along with the large intestine. This is where the body makes the decisions as to what is valuable to digest and absorb and what is waste.

When you're complete with that hold, walk your right index finger under the hand and over the thumb to the back of the left index finger, where it meets the thumb. At that juncture of bone is large intestine 4. This is also the point to massage if you've got a headache, but don't massage it if you're pregnant. Your thumb will slide across the inside of your wrist to lung 9, located on the inside wrist crease, just inside the thick tendon at the thumb side (figure 57). (You will feel a strong blood pulse here.)

Again, hold these points and visualize the organs of elimination. The lungs, filling the entire thoracic cavity, replace carbon dioxide with oxygen. The large intestine, connected to the small intestine and emptying its contents out the anus, further processes food and waste and removes solid waste from the system.

When you feel complete with that hold, curl your left middle finger over the right hand to triple warmer 4 and bring the left thumb onto circulation-sex 7, to begin the walk on the right hand now.

When you are complete, continue to sit still and feel the energy moving through your whole body.

Final Notes

By now you've seen that there are many ways to use Energy Medicine Yoga both in your daily yoga and as standalone practices. There are techniques that you can use in any pose, and the beauty of this practice is that you can customize it to fit your needs. Be experimental, be playful. Find what works for you.

Energy Medicine Yoga is a way of learning to listen to your body. You now know the places to thump, to tap, and to hold. You know how to weave your energy systems together. You know how to find the places where energy is stuck and how to massage it free. Get intimate with yourself. Feel the uniqueness of your body and all of its quirks. You will start to discover all the amazing, incredible, subtle ways the body communicates with you. You will be able to discover when it is getting sick, before the sickness takes hold. You'll be able to hear things when the body is still whispering, before it is forced to scream its messages.

I encourage you to listen and tune in to how you feel, both on a physical level and on an emotional and mental level. Get quiet and come into the present moment. Release the distractions of your daily life. Come into the center, come into neutral, where you release your desire for things to be one way or another and accept things just as they are. Then ask yourself: how does that feel? Learn and remember that feeling of neutral, that feeling of contentment and ease, so that you can come back to it again and again.

I also encourage you to get into the habit of doing some form of Energy Medicine Yoga every day, in the same way the groomers groom the ski mountain every single day. You don't have to do a ton, but do something. By now you've discovered that a little goes a long way. Build the positive habit fields. Build the positive energy connections. Get your energy habituated to waking up, to going in the right direction, to working with and for you. Except on the first days of your moon (menstrual) cycle or during a serious injury or illness, practice every day. Bring yourself to your mat and start to move.

And bring *all* of yourself to the mat. The part of you that is lazy or angry or tired. The part that is bored or disbelieving or disenchanted. When you are too busy, or when you are discontent, when your life is transcendent, and when it is falling apart, practice anyway. Come to the mat. Give yourself to the practice.

Life is a constant repetition of tasks. There is never completion. There are only more tasks—many of them the exact same tasks you did yesterday—washing dishes, doing laundry, making beds, cooking, eating, cleaning up. If you learn to enjoy the tasks and not the completion of the tasks, you can find happiness. But you must practice enjoying them, because the natural tendency is to long for the end of the task, to long for completion. In the same way, your Energy Medicine Yoga practice is, at first, the practice of enjoying the practices.

First you tap because the book tells you to tap. Then you start to feel a result from the tapping. You slowly do more and continue to try out new practices. After a while, using Energy Medicine Yoga techniques will become a habit, like brushing your teeth, and you wonder how you ever could have done without it. And then all of a sudden, your body is simply doing these practices because it knows them. You have become fluent in the language of your body. You have attained a level of mastery. You'll know you have reached that because if you start to do these practices daily, you'll feel it markedly when you skip a day or two. That is when Energy Medicine Yoga becomes the most potent—when you feel the need, the longing for the work.

Little by little, your practice will show you who you are, and it will be improving you, in every moment—not making you hotter, sexier, or slimmer, but allowing you to recognize your own divinity and your own humanity. You will increase your compassion for yourself and thereby increase it for others. You will feel yourself a part of the universe and begin to see the interconnection of everything. You will learn and discover things that I do not know and cannot write of here, because they will be your own secret mysteries. And your continual daily practice will also make you stronger, more flexible in body and mind, more resilient, calmer.

Your Energy Medicine Yoga practice will teach you to find the joy and presence of every moment. By devoting yourself to this work, you can discover your own inner strength, resilience, and intuition—the skills that will help you become the person that you truly are, powerful and potent in your own life, manifesting your desires, and content with your experiences. When you are deeply grounded, you can reach great heights. This practice will give you the tools to clear away the limitations that have been shrouding you. It will give you the courage and the willpower to follow your path. It will allow you to let the light of your soul shine forth.

Trauma and Energy Medicine Yoga

Because so many of us suffer from pain and grief and trauma—both large and small—that gets stored in our energy systems, I'm including here a primer on some easy ways to deal with and release them. This is a huge subject, but there are some simple tools I'd like to give you to help you start to dissipate these challenging energies, so you can experience more ease in your life.

There are many types of trauma. We can experience physical trauma, like a broken leg. We can experience emotional trauma, such as being fired from a job or losing a child. We can experience spiritual trauma, like a crisis of faith or a feeling of despair. And every type of trauma, not just physical, affects the body.

The energy of any trauma lives in the energetic fields of the body and in the chakras. It also lives in the tissues and cells of the body. Sometimes it appears in the physical body or the energetic body, and sometimes it appears in both. Sometimes the energy of nonphysical trauma can sit in the aura and slowly seep into the physical form, eventually causing physical problems. Emotional or residual physical trauma that is stuck in the physical body can increase over time and become denser, migrating from tissues into organs, hardening into stuck or frozen muscles or tumors.

However it appears and wherever it sits, trauma is disruptive. After the initial event that caused the trauma has ended, the body can relive it over and over again. In fact, this is the description of post-traumatic stress disorder (PTSD): The body is unable to distinguish real events from imagined events. If you have been traumatized and you think about the traumatic event, the same stress chemicals that were released into the body during the original event get released into the body as you think about it again. The body thinks the event is actually happening again and re-fires the same chemical and emotional response. This happens over and over, damaging the fragile nervous system, and causing stress to build up and imprint patterns in the body and the brain. Re-experiencing the body's reaction to the original trauma stops many people from being able to get past the event, integrate it in a healthy way, and move forward.

There are many books and studies linking the psychological and mind processes with the physical body. Louise Hay's wonderful book *Heal Your Body* lists some of the possible emotional components to a physical ailment. She uses positive affirmations to help release the physical disease. But often, because of the habits maintained in our body's energy fields, "wishing yourself well" isn't enough.

One of the main purposes of any type of yoga, including Energy Medicine Yoga, is to keep the body supple and flexible. The body holds memories and emotions in its physical form. Many yoga teachers talk about the sexual or family issues held in the hips. Struggles with finances and feeling overburdened by life are said to be held in the back. Troubles with the neck point to our stubbornness or inflexibility on issues.

The more open and flexible the body is, the more open and flexible the mind can be. Opening up space in the body allows the energy of stuck, deeply held emotions to move and be released.

The problem is, while experiencing an emotional release from, say, a deep hip opener or backbend, can feel cathartic, it can also feel terrifying. And if you are dealing with a trauma like sexual abuse or deep grief, it can feel overwhelming.

In part 1, I talked about the frontal neurovascular points on the forehead. These "Oh my God!" points are among the most powerful tools you can use to help reprogram your nervous system and keep it from going into stress response at the memory of a traumatic experience. I use those points constantly during my yoga practice. Sometimes I use them to diffuse the energy of trauma, and sometimes I use them just to keep myself more present and focused in a pose.

If you are in a yoga class and starting to have an emotional release (or if you are anywhere and starting to have an emotional release), immediately put one hand over your forehead. You can also put both hands over your forehead and your thumbs on your temples, which is a triple warmer point. You can also cover your eyes with your palms and let your fingers come up over your forehead into your hairline, like we did in the palming exercise in the eye yoga chapter.

All of these holds help to calm the nervous system, keep blood in the forebrain, and interrupt the fight-or-flight response. They allow the story to occur without the emotional charge of the story. The longer you hold these points while the story runs through your mind, the more the charge dissipates.

You can do the same thing intentionally, as well, to diffuse old trauma. Bring up the difficult story while holding these points. This interrupts the flow of energy to the limbic system of the brain and stops the stress response from sending out the cascade of stress hormones. The story doesn't go away, but the physiological response to it lessens and lessens until it becomes just a story, just a part of your history, not something that triggers you into a full emotional meltdown.

You can use those hand positions in almost any yoga pose, but especially those where you are on your belly and returning your head to the floor. I rest my head in my hands every time I release my head back to the floor in belly poses. It is wonderfully calming and nurturing and allows your head to completely release all its static and clutter. I like to hold my forehead in forward bends too. If you're less flexible and can't bring your arms or elbows to the floor in a forward bend, use a bolster or block to rest your arms on, so you can reach your hands to your head.

Holding the triple warmer neurovascular point in the throat hollow also calms the nervous system. I use this point often when I'm on the phone with someone challenging or when I'm in the car and someone cuts me off in traffic. Holding this point has the effect of immediately bringing you back to balance and clarity. You can hold this point in many poses, which is why I use the triple warmer/heart mudra for all the prayer positions.

The book *The Promise of Energy Psychology*, by David Feinstein, PhD; Donna Eden; and Gary Craig, teaches the Emotional Freedom Technique (EFT) for discharging trauma. EFT has been used to great effect with veterans suffering from PTSD. It uses tapping, and as you know, tapping speaks to the body in its own language. When you feel an emotional wave start to engulf you, tap successively on the following points:

- the outside of the eyes
- between the eyes, at the edges of the eyebrows
- directly under the eyes
- under the nose
- under the lower lip
- K-27
- the thymus
- the spleen points on the side seams of the body
- the outside edges of your thighs, where the fingers naturally land if your arms are at your sides
- the outer edge of the hand—the karate-chop side

The research on why these particular points work is related to the connection of these major meridian points to the amygdala, the part of the brain responsible for activating and remembering emotional distress. Tapping on these points interrupts the flow of electrical energy to the amygdala at the same time you're remembering the traumatic event. This interruption changes the flow of the neural pathways.

The Promise of Energy Psychology also has many poses useful for activating the radiant circuits, which can help diffuse trauma by increasing joy.

If you are struggling with deep trauma, I encourage you to seek professional help. There is no need to suffer alone with trauma, and many resources are out there to help you.

RESOURCES

Innersource (innersource.net), website for Donna Eden and Eden Energy Medicine.

ParaYoga (parayoga.com), website for Rod Stryker and ParaYoga.

The Gold Standard for EFT (emofree.com), website for Gary Craig and the Emotional Freedom Technique.

The Succulence Revolution (thesucculencerevolution.com), resources for sacred women practices mentioned in the "Special Note to Women" near the end of the bandha section (see week 3).

Lauren K. Walker: Writer, Teacher, Yogi (lkwalker.com), website for Lauren Walker and her work.

angela-victor.com, website for Angela Farmer.

Jivamukti (jivamuktiyoga.com), website for Jivamukti and co-founder David Life.

LifeSpa® (lifespa.com), website for Dr. John Douillard and Ayurvedic research.

BIBLIOGRAPHY

Aja. "Sanskrit: The Language of the Gods." Atma Institute, n.d. atmainstitute.org/sanskrit.htm.

Bowditch, Bruce. "Prana Vayu: Five Vital Forces." *Yoga* (blog). July 3, 2008. sacred-earth.typepad.com/yoga/2008/07/prana-vayu-five-vital-forces.html.

Craig, Gary, Donna Eden, and David Feinstein, PhD. *The Promise of Energy Psychology.* New York: Tarcher/Penguin, 2005.

Desikachar, T. K. V. *The Heart of Yoga: Developing a Personal Practice.* Rochester, VT: Inner Traditions, 1995.

Desilets, Saida, PhD. *Emergence of the Sensual Woman.* Kihei, HI: Jade Goddess Publishing, 2006.

Diamond, John, MD. *Life Energy: Using the Meridians to Unlock the Hidden Power of Your Emotions.* New York: Paragon House, 1985.

Eden, Donna, with David Feinstein, PhD. *Energy Medicine.* New York: Penguin Putnam Inc., 1998.

Eden, Donna, with David Feinstein, PhD. *Energy Medicine for Women.* New York: Jeremy P. Tarcher/ Penguin, 2008.

Fallon, Sally, with Mary G. Enig, PhD. *Nourishing Traditions: The Cookbook that Challenges Politically Correct Nutrition and the Diet Dictocrats.* Washington, DC: New Trends Publishing, 1999.

Feuerstein, Georg, PhD. *The Yoga Tradition: Its History, Literature, Philosophy and Practice.* Prescott, AZ: Hohm Press, 1998.

Forrest, Ana T. *Fierce Medicine.* New York: HarperOne, 2011.

Frawley, David, Dr. *Tantric Yoga and the Wisdom Goddesses.* Twin Lakes, WI: Lotus Press, 2003.

Frawley, David, Dr., Dr. Avinash Lele, and Dr. Subhash Ranade. *Ayurveda and Marma Therapy: Energy Points in Yogic Healing.* Twin Lakes, WI: Lotus Press, 2012.

Grossman, Marc, O.D., L.Ac., and Vinton McCabe, N.V.E. *Greater Vision: A Comprehensive Program for Physical, Emotional, and Spiritual Clarity.* Los Angeles: Keats Publishing, 2001.

Hay, Louise L. *Heal Your Body.* Carson, CA: Hay House, 1982.

Hirschi, Gertrude. *Mudras: Yoga in Your Hands.* San Francisco: Red Wheel/ Weiser, LLC, 2000.

Jawahir, Dylan. "The Soleus Muscle, the Second Heart." *August Point Wellness Center* (blog). May 25, 2012. augustpoint.wordpress.com/2012/05/25/the-soleus-muscle-the-second-heart/.

Kapit, Wynn, and Lawrence M. Elson. *The Anatomy Coloring Book.* New York: Addison-Wesley Educational Publishers, Inc., 1993.

Lipton, Bruce, PhD. *The Biology of Belief.* Santa Rosa, CA: Mountain of Love/Elite Books, 2005.

Macdonell, Arthur Anthony, MA, PhD, Hon. L.L.D.A. *A Practical Sanskrit Dictionary.* New Delhi, India: Munshiram Manoharlal Publishers, 1999.

McCall, Timothy, MD. *Yoga as Medicine.* New York: Bantam Dell, 2007.

Ober, Clinton, Stephen T. Sinatra, and Martin Zucker. *Earthing: The Most Important Health Discovery Ever?* Laguna Beach, CA: Basic Health Publications, 2010.

Onofrio, Karen R., MD. *What's Under Your Skin: Practical Anatomy for Eden Energy Medicine Practitioners.* Self-published.

Parry, Danaan. *Warriors of the Heart.* Cooperstown, NY: Sunstone Publications, 1991.

Saraswati, Swami Satyananda. *Yoga Nidra.* Bihar, India: Bihar School of Yoga, 1998.

Satchidananda, Yogiraj Sri Swami. *Integral Yoga Hatha.* Buckingham, VA: Integral Yoga Publications, 1995.

Schneider, Meir. *Yoga for Your Eyes.* Boulder, CO: Sounds True, 1999.

Showkeir, Jamie, and Maren Showkeir. *Yoga Wisdom at Work.* San Francisco: Berrett-Koehler Publishers, 2013.

Snyder, Kimberly, CN. *The Beauty Detox Foods.* Harlequin Books, 2013.

Stryker, Rod. *The Four Desires.* New York: Delacorte Press, 2011.

Takahashi, Takeo. *Atlas of the Human Body.* New York: Harper Perennial, 1989.

Tigunait, Pandit Rajmani, PhD. *The Power of Mantra and the Mystery of Initiation.* Honesdale, PA: Himalayan Institute Press, 1996.

Tsiaras, Alexander, and Barry Werth. *The Architecture and Design of Man and Woman.* New York: Doubleday, 2004.

Young, Emma. "Gut Instincts: The Secrets of Your Second Brain." *New Scientist* 216 (December, 2012): 38–42. Reproduced at *Neuroscience* (blog); December 18, 2012. neurosciencestuff.tumblr.com/post/38271759345/gut-instincts-the-secrets-of-your-second-brain.

ACKNOWLEDGMENTS

Energy Medicine Yoga is a synthesis of many techniques I've studied over the years. However, there are two that are the most important and most influential on my own practice and teaching.

The first is ParaYoga. I've been studying with ParaYoga founder Rod Stryker since 2000 and was initiated into the lineage in 2007. This ancient, methodical, spiritual, and scientific approach to yoga has been a wellspring of solace and power for me. The inclusion of deep meditation practices, visualization, and articulate asana, as well as devotion to prayer, mantra, and guru, have allowed me to enter a world of yoga previously unknown to me. My initiation into the lineage further melted my attachment to ego, allowing me ever-deeper access to the profound techniques of ParaYoga. I bow down at the lotus feet of my teacher, Yogarupa, and his teacher, and his teacher's teachers.

The second most profound synthesis of ideas I've discovered is Eden Energy Medicine. Founded by Donna Eden, Eden Energy Medicine (EEM) supports and heals hundreds of thousands of people worldwide with its simple, powerful, and accessible techniques. Based on the truth that energy is all there is, EEM practitioners begin to work with their own basic essential nature at its source: vibration and energy. My devotion and love for Donna are unbounded. Her unconditional support and openhearted generosity are a rare gift to this world, and I am not alone in considering her a living master.

It is very powerful to have both of these teachers present in the synthesis practice of Energy Medicine Yoga, because this yoga system is both the masculine and the feminine, the yin and the yang. In order for us to become whole and healthy beings in this world, we have to balance these elements within ourselves. I find it particularly interesting that until both of these teachers appeared in my life, I was not able to truly move forward with my own dharma. Once again, the universe was at play, bringing powerful feminine and masculine energies together to teach me something that is more than a sum of its parts.

Although writing is a very solitary practice, the creation of a book is a group effort. My endless thanks go out to all the people who have helped me along the way with encouragement, material and spiritual support, and succor, and for holding strong the belief that what I was doing with my life was going to be valuable both to myself and others, even when it may not have appeared to be so.

My mother has unwaveringly supported me through a long and often strange-looking career path, always championing my unique, out-of-the-box approach, never asking me to be more "normal." I will never be able to thank her enough for her love and confidence in me. To my dad, who I only ever wanted to make proud: I'm doing your work in the world—I am a teacher and a writer. I love you endlessly for your faith in me. My sister, Jennifer, has provided me with more insight and wisdom, truth telling, and love than even she knows, as well as being the best first pair of eyes and yoga tech for this whole book.

I'm forever indebted to Michael and Leslie Gaffin for their unequivocal support and love, and the space to write the first draft of *Energy Medicine Yoga*. To Kristy Gange for introducing me to Donna's work and forever changing my life. To PJ de Groot for showing me the power of Donna's work and helping me to be a better writer. And an enormous debt of thanks and gratitude to Ann Hood, for helping to make me a real writer in the first place.

Thank you to my students at Norwich University for making me a better teacher and helping to birth *Energy Medicine Yoga*. Thank you to Colonel Michael Kelley, former commandant of cadets, for his unwavering trust that yoga would help the cadets and for spearheading our yoga study. Thank you Vermont Student Assistance Corporation for your generous financial support of my studies of Eden Energy Medicine. A huge thank you to Titanya Dahlin for insisting I finally take the EEM certified practitioner program and for seeding the idea of this book, to Dondi Dahlin for her incredible support and encouraging me to write it, to David Feinstein for his wisdom, grace, unending help, and true friendship.

My profound gratitude goes to the entire team at Innersource. A special thanks to Roger Devenyns; to all the teachers at Innersource, especially Susan Stone, Lisa Buford, Sara Allen, Kelmie Blake, Amy McDowell, Camille Pipolo, and Donna Kemper; and to all my co-students in the EEM certified practitioner program, especially Meredith Mills. Thank you to Maria Petrova for tensegrity. Thank you to the brilliant Dr. James Oschman and Dr. Bruce Lipton, for their incredible insights that are changing how we think about the world.

My thanks to Eileen McKusick, who helped me understand sound and healing in the aura and for our barefoot walks comparing notes on this process of writing our books. Thank you to all my fellow Para Yogis, especially Tracee Stanley. Thank you to my amazing friends and co-travelers on the path who were instrumental in keeping me in balance and joy as this book birthed: Elaine Doll, Liza Taylor, Mary Person, Jennifer Micheletti, Paula Koch. Thank you TB Gray for the groomer rides. To my second mom and biggest teacher, Dora Silver, my love and gratitude are yours.

At Sounds True I found the best publishing family I ever could have hoped for. Thank you, Jennifer Brown, for everything! Amy Rost is the best editor I could have imagined, pushing me to produce my best work and telling me when I got there. Thank you to Steven Lessard, Drummond West, Hayden Peltier, Aron Arnold, and Kasmah McDermott. Thank you to Lisa Kerans and the whole art department for making this book beautiful. Thank you to Dee Sandella and Michael Myers. Thank you to Matt Samet, Leslie Brown, and Haven Iverson. Thanks to the marketing and publicity team and all the players who helped get this book into the hands of so many people, especially Wendy Gardner, Lisa Trank, and Tucker Collins.

Thank you to David Life, my first yoga teacher, who showed me the true power of yoga. Thank you to my teacher trainer, Swami Ramananda, who was the first one to see the teacher in me.

I bow down at the lotus feet of all my yoga and spiritual teachers.

And my biggest thank you of all goes to my students, who will always be my best teachers! I bow down at your lotus feet in endless gratitude.

ABOUT THE AUTHOR

Lauren Walker has been teaching yoga and meditation since 1997. She splits her time between New England and Montana. A writer since childhood, Lauren publishes widely and has written features for the *New York Times,* the *Jerusalem Post,* and Salon.com. She has a periodic yoga column at MNN.com and has been featured in *Yoga Journal.* Lauren is a wandering spirit, and has lived and worked all over the world. She continues to travel and teach workshops and classes in the United States, Canada, and abroad. She is also a composer, hockey player, avid skier, and primitive-skills enthusiast. For more on Lauren and Energy Medicine Yoga, please visit lkwalker.com.

ABOUT SOUNDS TRUE

Sounds True is a multimedia publisher whose mission is to inspire and support personal transformation and spiritual awakening. Founded in 1985 and located in Boulder, Colorado, we work with many of the leading spiritual teachers, thinkers, healers, and visionary artists of our time. We strive with every title to preserve the essential "living wisdom" of the author or artist. It is our goal to create products that not only provide information to a reader or listener, but that also embody the quality of a wisdom transmission.

For those seeking genuine transformation, Sounds True is your trusted partner. At SoundsTrue.com you will find a wealth of free resources to support your journey, including exclusive weekly audio interviews, free downloads, interactive learning tools, and other special savings on all our titles.

To learn more, please visit SoundsTrue.com/bonus/free_gifts or call us toll free at 800-333-9185.

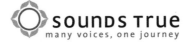

SOUNDS TRUE
many voices, one journey